# Ace the PCCN®!

You can do it!

Study Guide

Nicole Kupchik

MN, RN, CCNS, CCRN-K, PCCN-K

Nicole Kupchik Consulting, Inc.

Seattle, WA

Ace the PCCN®! Study Guide



Nicole Kupchik Consulting and Education

ISBN-10: 0-9978349-3-5

ISBN-13: 978-0-9978349-3-2

Cover design by O'Daniel Designs

Printed in the United States of America

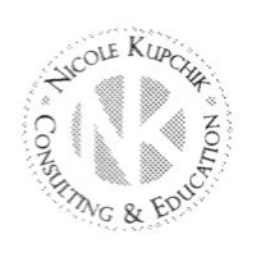


Seattle, WA

www.nicolekupchikconsulting.com

# Special thanks...

To my husband, Carl

My mom, Carol, who passed away in 2019

My many awesome friends
(you all know who you are)

Dr. Elizabeth Bridges, for your years of mentoring

Gina O'Daniel for her creative cover design

My colleagues at Harborview & Swedish who
have always encouraged me over the years!

And the THOUSANDS of nurses who have attended
my classes, given constructive feedback and taken
the exams! You are all an inspiration to me!

The encouragement you all have given me is
immeasurable and completely appreciated!

# Foreword

The Institute of Medicine's landmark report the *Future of Nursing* issued a call for nurses to lead, including nursing leadership at the point of care.[1] While we often think about leadership as a position, it has another definition. **A leader is "an expert clinician, involved in providing direct clinical care, who influences others to continuously improve the care they provide."** [2]

One key aspect to providing this leadership is clinical expertise and the ability to use evidence to inform practice. Preparation for certification is more than the rote memorization of facts. It is about teasing out complex situations and identifying critical information to guide your practice. The process of preparing for certification will advance your knowledge, competence and understanding the complexities of critical care nursing. [3]

But equally important to the increase in overt knowledge, this process will have less obvious or conceptual effects, such as an increased awareness of the evidence that support your practice, an increased confidence in your ability and passion to use evidence culminating

---

1 Institute of Medicine Committee on the Robert Wood Johnson Foundation Initiative on the Future of Nursing at IoM. The Future of Nursing: Leading Change, Advancing Health. Washington (DC): *National Academies Press* (US); 2011.

2 Cook MJ. Improving care requires leadership in nursing. *Nurse Educ Today*. 1999;19(4):306-12.

3 Sayre C, Wyant S, Karvonen C. Effect of a medical-surgical practice and certification review course on clinical nursing practice. *J Nurs Staff Dev*. 2010;26(1):11-6.

in the "aha" moments when concepts come to life. Ultimately this subtle and empowering use of evidence supports its more overt or instrumental use, to persuade others and to advocate for practice and policy change. [4,5]

How do these concepts apply to this book? *Ace the PCCN!* is a book designed to help you gain knowledge and enhance your ability to interpret and respond to complex clinical situations. But this book is not just a resource to aid you in preparing for a certification examination. Rather it reflects the author's passion to support your development as an expert progressive care and telemetry nurse. Along the way, the process towards certification may enhance both your conceptual and instrumental use of evidence. Think back to the definition of leadership, this journey to certification is really a journey to leadership and the advancement of our profession, and that is exactly what Nicole Kupchik is committed to.

—Elizabeth Bridges
PhD, RN, CCNS, FCCM, FAAN

4 Nutley S, Walter I, Davies H. How research can inform public services. Bristol, UK: *The Policy Press*, 2007.

5 Wilkinson JE. *Impacts of evidence use-hard hitting or subtle change? Worldviews on Evidence-Based Nursing.* 2010;7(1):1-3.

Unless we are making
progress in our nursing
every year, every month, every week,
take my word for it,
we are going back.

—Florence Nightingale (May 1872)

# Contents

You can do it!

# A note of encouragement from Nicole...

Congratulations on taking steps to becoming certified and obtaining the PCCN®!

In 2002, I passed the CCRN® for the first time. I am going to let you in on a little secret. I was eligible to sit the exam in 1994. I attended three certification review courses before taking the exam. Why? I lacked confidence and was so afraid of failing! I finally got up the courage in 2002 and aced it!

I can distinctly remember walking out of the testing site questioning myself, wondering why I waited so long to take it! I had so much self-doubt. It was a little crazy, because clinically, I knew my stuff! A couple years later, I started teaching sections of the exam at Harborview Medical Center and in 2006 started co-teaching the combo CCRN® & PCCN® prep courses nationally.

Who would think someone could go from having a complete lack of confidence to teaching the courses a few years later?! Mental mindset is everything. I want you to tell yourself every day that you can do this!!!

I often hear nurses say "becoming certified doesn't make you a better nurse". I completely disagree with statements like this. The journey you will take in preparing to become certified increases your knowledge to better care for your patients. I truly believe every nurse should be certified in their specialty.

I was inspired to publish this book by nurses who have attended my review courses. Many of the study books available are overwhelming & contain too much information. My goal is always to break down disease states into digestible pieces so you learn! The book is written with the purpose of being succinct & easy to read with bullet point formatting.

My biggest piece of advice to you in studying is, of course to understand different conditions, but do as many practice test questions as possible. Read rationales for questions you get right & those you miss. Consider using Ace the PCCN®: You can do it! Practice Question Review book to assist. The book contains 3 full practice tests and all answers have rationales. I believe practicing test questions is the key to success!

# About the PCCN® Exam

The PCCN® is administered by the American Association of Critical Care Nurses (AACN). Website: www.aacn.org

## Qualifications to sit the exam:

- Hold a current unencumbered nursing license
- Practice 1,750 hours in the previous 2 years
- 875 hours in the most recent year preceding application
- RNs or APRNs practicing > 5 years with at least 2,000 practice hours, only need to work 144 hours in the most recent year
- If you have any questions about eligibility, please contact AACN—they are super helpful!

The application consists of 3 pages total. Two pages ask about demographic data, one page is an honor statement. You will need to provide the name & contact information of a colleague or manager who can verify your eligibility.

Once AACN receives your application, they usually take about 2 - 3 weeks for processing. Once it has been processed & you are deemed eligible, you will receive communication from a company called AMP/PSI. They will give you directions to schedule your exam. You have 90 days to take your exam. Easy peasy!

The PCCN® exam consists of 125 questions. Twenty five questions will not count toward your final score. They are used for statistical data for future exams. It's kind of a bummer that you don't know which ones don't count. The advice I ALWAYS give nurses—if you come across a question that you have NO idea the answer, tell yourself it's a question that doesn't count! Don't psych yourself out if you don't know the answer. There will be some questions that you just don't know.

Exam questions are written at the application & analysis levels based on Synergy model of care; meaning they aren't basic questions. They want to know you know how to take care of patients and what to anticipate in treatment. On that same thought, they also aren't trying to trick you. Each question will have 4 answer choices and only one is the correct answer.

You will have 3 hours to complete the exam. The passing "cut score" is 68. You have to get 68 correct out of 100. Translated—you have to score about 68% correct to pass. That's it!!! You can do this!!!! BUT, you have to go in prepared. The reported pass rate for the PCCN® exam is about 75%. The way they score is a little more complicated than a straight 68%, but I'm not completely sure exactly how that's done! You can do this!!!

**THE PCCN® TEST PLAN**
**UPDATED IN 2019**

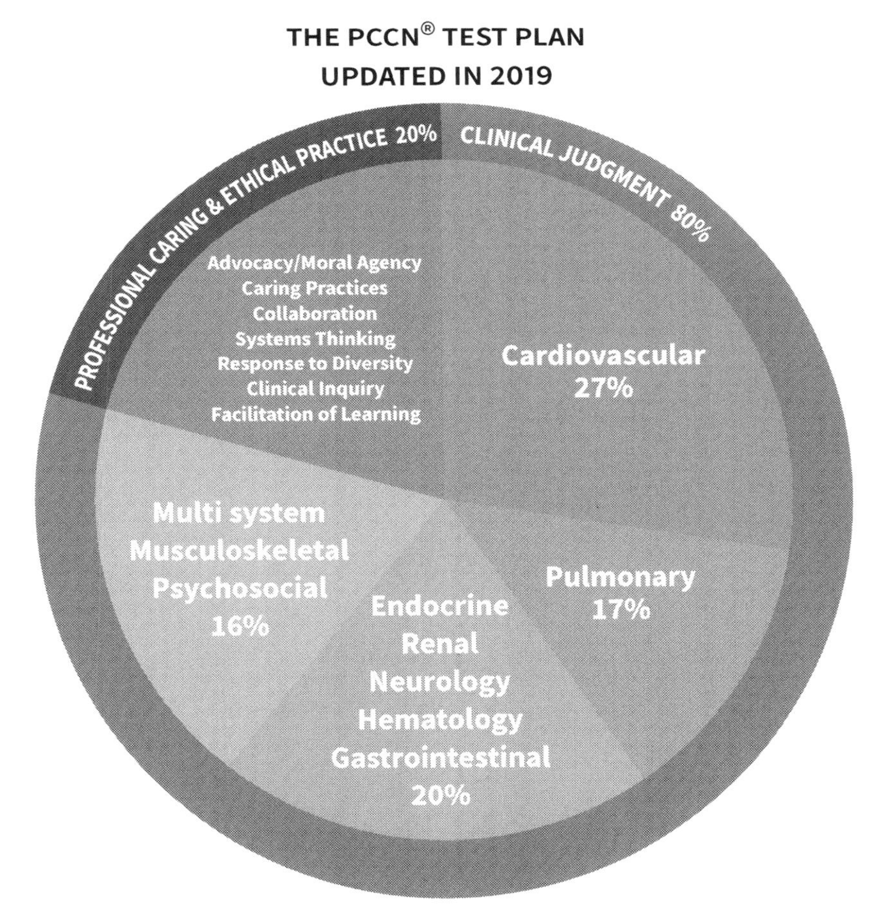

**GENERAL TEST TIPS:**

- ✓ Go in with a confident attitude! You can do this!
- ✓ Get to the testing site on time
- ✓ Answer every question
- ✓ You can change answers, but...DON'T!!
- ✓ You'll have a clock on the bottom of your computer screen
- ✓ Pace yourself
- ✓ You will find out right away if you passed!

Positive Mental Attitude

You Can Do It!

# Cardiovascular Review

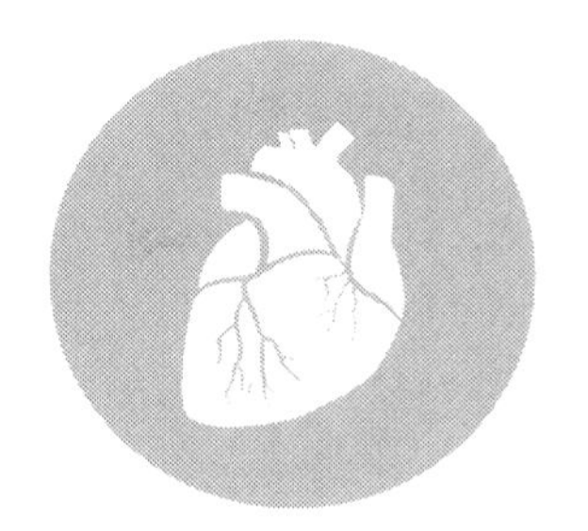

## AACN Test Plan for the Cardiovascular portion of the PCCN® Exam

- Acute coronary syndromes
  - Non-ST segment elevation myocardial infarction
  - ST segment elevation myocardial infarction
  - Unstable angina
- Acute inflammatory disease (e.g., myocarditis, endocarditis, pericarditis)
- Aneurysm – Dissection & repair
- Cardiac surgery (post ICU care)
- Cardiac tamponade
- Cardiac/vascular Catheterization – diagnostic/interventional
- Cardiogenic shock
- Cardiomyopathies
  - Dilated (e.g., ischemic/non-ischemic), stress-induced (e.g., Takotsubo)
  - Hypertrophic
- Dysrhythmias
- Heart failure - acute exacerbations (e.g., pulmonary edema), chronic
- Hypertension – uncontrolled
- Hypertensive crisis
- Minimally invasive cardiac surgery (i.e., non-sternal approach)
- Valvular heart disease
- Vascular disease

# Coronary Artery Perfusion

- Both the right & left **coronary arteries** arise at the base of the aorta (Sinus of Valsalva); immediately above the aortic valve
- Coronary arteries are perfused during diastole

# Heart Sounds

## Valvular auscultation points:

- Aortic valve: Right sternal border, 2nd ICS
- Pulmonic valve: Left sternal border, 2nd ICS
- Tricuspid valve: Left sternal border, 4 - 5th ICS
- Mitral valve: Left mid-clavicular line, 5th ICS

## Normal Heart Sounds

- **$S_1$**: closure of the mitral & tricuspid valves
  - Loudest over mitral area, 5th ICS
  - Systole
  - 1/3 of the cardiac cycle
- **$S_2$**: closure of pulmonic & aortic valve
  - Loudest over aortic area, 2nd ICS
  - Diastole
  - 2/3 of the cardiac cycle

## Extra Heart Sounds

- **$S_3$**: Ventricular gallop
  - Auscultated in fluid overload; when preload is elevated
  - Normal in kids, high cardiac output, 3rd trimester of pregnancy
  - Listen over apex area
  - Sound is caused by a rapid rush of blood into a dilated, overfilled ventricle
  - Other causes: Cardiomyopathy, ventricular septal defect (VSD), mitral or tricuspid regurgitation

- $S_4$: Atrial gallop (pre-systolic)
  - Sound caused by vibration of atria ejecting into non-compliant ventricles
  - Auscultated during ischemia (increased resistance to ventricular filling)
  - Other causes: Ischemia, HTN, pulmonary stenosis, CAD, aortic stenosis, left ventricular hypertrophy
  - Listen over tricuspid or mitral area
- Split Heart Sounds
  - When one valve closes later than the other
    - **Best heard during *inspiration*
  - Split $S_1$—Mitral closes before tricuspid valve
    - RBBB, PVCs, ventricular pacing
  - Split $S_2$—Aortic closes before pulmonic valve
    - Overfilled right ventricle
    - Atrial septal defect (ASD)

# Acute Coronary Syndrome

**Pathophysiology:** Progressive atherosclerosis with plaque rupture causing blood clot formation leading to an imbalance of $O_2$ supply & demand

## In ACS, there is an imbalance of oxygen supply & demand

### $O_2$ Supply:

- Coronary arteries
- Diastolic filling time
- Cardiac output
- Hemoglobin
- $SaO_2/SpO_2$

### $O_2$ Demand:

- Heart rate
- Contractility
- Preload
- Afterload

## Cardiac Risk Factors

### Non-modifiable:

- » Age
- » Gender
- » Family history
- » Race

### Modifiable:

- » Smoking
- » Hyperlipidemia
- » Obesity
- » Diabetes mellitus
- » Diet
- » Physical inactivity
- » Hypertension

## Cardiac Biomarkers:

- » Troponin I (or T) is the most sensitive & specific
- » Elevates in 3 - 6 hours
- » Peaks in 14 - 20 hours
- » Returns to normal in 1 - 2 weeks
- » Most labs > 0.4 mcg/L is considered elevated
- » CPK, CK-MB & myoglobin may also be elevated
  - No longer recommended to routinely check

## Unstable Angina & Non-ST Elevation MI (NSTE-ACS)

### Chest pain assessment—ask these questions:

- » **O**nset?
- » **L**ocation?
- » **D**uration?
- » **C**haracteristics?
- » **A**ssociated s/s?
- » **R**elieving factors?
- » **T**reatment?

*Reminder: Women and diabetics may have atypical presentation

## Angina

- Stable
  - Exertional; Symptoms cease when exertion stops
  - May have a fixed vessel stenosis with demand ischemia
  - May require sublingual nitroglycerin
- Unstable (UA)
  - Increasing frequency, time & duration
  - Sign & precursor to a MI
  - 10 – 20% have a MI
  - May consider anti-platelet therapy
- Variant (Prinzmetal's)
  - Sudden pain caused from coronary artery vasospasm
  - Occurs at rest or when sleeping
  - Get 12 lead ECG with & without symptoms!
  - Will see ECG changes with pain and symptoms
  - Treat with nitroglycerin (NTG) and calcium channel blockers to relieve spasm

## NON-ST Elevation ACS (NSTE-ACS)

- Partial occlusion of coronary artery
- Pain/symptoms may occur at rest & last > 20 min
- Hallmark sign—pain with ↑ frequency, heaviness or pressure
- 12 lead ECG: ST depression or T wave inversion (ischemia)
- 8 or more leads with ST depression/T wave inversion & ST elevation in aVR, high suspicion for proximal LAD occlusion
- Cardiac biomarkers elevated
- Treatment: PCI; early PCI if high risk

## ST Elevation MI (STEMI)

- Complete occlusion of a coronary artery
- Emergency! Activate the Cath Lab!
- 12 lead ECG: ST elevation (infarction)
- Hallmark signs—Chest pain or pressure > 20 min, SOB, diaphoresis
- Causes: Plaque rupture leading to blood clot formation
  - Platelets aggregate to the atherosclerotic site/ plaque rupture

- Other causes: coronary vessel dissection, fixed coronary lesion, cocaine
- Occlusive thrombus formation

» + Cardiac biomarkers

» Treatment: Immediate reperfusion

- Cath lab for PCI (preferred) or
- If Cath lab is not readily available—fibrinolytics, then Cath lab as soon as possible

**ST depression** = ischemia

**ST elevation** = injury

» ≥ 1 mm in limb leads (I, II, III, aVF, aVL) or ≥ 2 mm in precordial leads ($V_1$–$V_6$) and/or

» New left BBB precordial leads

» In 2 or more contiguous leads

- Leads that look at the same wall of the heart

## Timing of ECG Changes in STEMI:

» **Immediate:** T wave elevation, ST ↑ in leads over the area of infarction

» **Within a few hours:** Large upright T waves

» **Several hours:** After revascularization, ST normalizes, T waves invert

» **Several hours–days:** Q waves may develop, reduced R waves, low voltage R wave (sometimes for life)

## Emergent STEMI Treatment:

### Aspirin

» 81 mg – 325 mg PO load—chewed!

- Rectal may be used if unable to take PO

» Onset of action 1 – 7.5 min

» Inhibits cyclooxygenase-1 within platelets → prevents formation of thromboxane $A_2$

» Disables platelet aggregation

» Monitor for intolerance and bleeding

» Used indefinitely post MI

» Maintenance dose for life at least 81 mg daily

## Nitroglycerin (NTG)

- 0.4 mg SL every 5 minutes x 3
- Sublingual, spray or infusion (Tridil)
- May use IV if continued chest discomfort/symptoms
- Potent vasodilator
- Monitor for hypotension, headache
- Reduces preload & ventricular wall tension
- Decreases myocardial $O_2$ consumption
- Avoid if suspected right ventricular infarction or use of phosphodiesterase (PDE) inhibitors (Viagra or Cialis)

## Supplemental $O_2$ only if sats < 94%

- Hyperoxemia perpetuates oxidative injury after MI
    - Can worsen and ↑ infarct size
- Not needed for patients without evidence of respiratory distress (AHA guideline)

## Morphine

- Small incremental doses IV Q 5 - 15 min if chest pain is unrelieved by NTG
- Use as adjunct therapy to NTG
- Potent analgesic & anxiolytic
- Causes venodilation & reduces preload, mild afterload reduction
- Decreases workload of heart
- Use cautiously in UA & NSTEMI!!
    - Increased mortality in a large patient registry
    - Causes hypotension
- Avoid if suspected right ventricular infarction

## Post PCI therapy, consider:

- Access site management
  - Radial artery access site is becoming more popular; fewer complications
    - Monitor for arterial vasospasm
  - Femoral—monitor for bleeding, hematoma, retroperitoneal bleeding
    - Rare cases, can develop pseudoaneurysms, A/V fistula
- Retroperitoneal bleeding—will see "soft" BP that is fluid responsive
  - Back pain
  - Tachycardia
    - May not see if patient received beta blockers
  - Late sign is flank ecchymosis (Grey-Turner's sign)
  - Assess coags
  - Control bleeding
- Monitor renal function closely (secondary to dye load)

## Post-PCI medication management:

### Post MI with PCI, patients are prescribed "The Big 5"

1) Aspirin (indefinitely)
2) P2Y12 Inhibitor (usually for 1 year)
3) Beta Blocker (indefinitely)
4) Statin (high dose indefinitely)
5) ACE Inhibitor or ARB (If EF < 40%, indefinitely)

### Dual Anti-Platelet Therapy for at least 1 year post PCI

- **Aspirin** (indefinitely) **plus**
- **Thienopyridines** ($P_2Y_{12}$ Inhibitors)—**with drug eluting stents (DES) or bare metal stents (BMS):**
  - Clopidogrel (Plavix) 300 - 600 mg load; continue 75 mg daily for 12 months **or**
  - Prasugrel (Effient) 60 mg load; continue 10 mg for 12 months **or**
  - Brilinta (Ticagreolor) 180 mg load; 90 mg BID for 12 months
  - Drug duration shorter w/BMS

## On a case by case basis, the Cardiology provider may prescribe:

- Unfractionated Heparin (UFH) **or**
- Bivalirudin (Angiomax®)—used during PCI; finish in Cath lab
  - Half-life is 25 min with normal renal function

  Dose:
  - 0.75 mg/kg IV bolus
  - Then 1.75 mg/kg/hr IV infusion for duration of the procedure
  - May continue for 4 hours post procedure
- GP IIb/IIIa Inhibitors (at time of PCI)
  - Abciximab (Reopro)
  - Eptifibatide (Integrilin)
  - Tirofiban (Aggrastat)
    - Monitor platelet count
    - Monitor for bleeding!

# Other medications:

## Beta Blockers: "-olols"

- Start within 24° if hemodynamically stable
- Hold if hypotension or signs of hypoperfusion/shock
- Metoprolol tartrate & carvedilol mostly used
  - Metoprolol tartrate is the only form of metoprolol that is cardio-protective!
- Blocks catecholamine & sympathetic nervous system
- Cardio-protective, decreases arrhythmias
- Decreases HR & contractility
- Decreases myocardial $O_2$ consumption
- Long term, decreases morbidity & mortality
- Continued indefinitely
- Educate patients on symptoms, may feel exhausted, depressed

## Statins (HMG CoA Reductase Inhibitors)

- ↓ cholesterol levels by interfering with body's ability to produce cholesterol
- ↓ inflammatory response that theoretically may be responsible for atherosclerotic process
- Cardio-protective
- Decreases risk of recurrent MI and stroke
- High-dose recommended for all post MI patients with:
  - Atorvastatin (Lipitor), rosuvastatin (Crestor), lovastatin (Mevacor), or simvastatin (Zocor)
  - Monitor for muscle myopathies & myositis
- Target LDL < 70
  - May exacerbate Type 2 diabetes
  - Monitor LFTs
  - Rhabdomyolysis—extremely rare

## ACE Inhibitors ("prils") or Angiotensin Receptor Blockers ("sartans")

- Used if EF < 40%, new heart failure
- ↓ Intra-cardiac pressures
- Prevents cardiac remodeling
- ↓ Preload & afterload

**Common ARBs:**

Valsartan (Diovan),
Losartan (Cozaar, Candesartan, Olmesartan)

**Common ACE Inhibitors:**

Ramipril (Altace)
Lisinopril (Zestril, Prinivil)
Enalapril (Vasotec)
Captopril (Capoten)

## Side Effects of ACE-Inhibitors & ARBs:

- Cough – 19%! (Don't see with ARBs)
  - ACE Inhibitors prevent the breakdown of bradykinin & substance P in the lungs
  - Accumulation of protussive mediators
  - Can use ARB instead
- Hypotension
  - 1st dose effect
  - Syncope & dizziness
- Hyperkalemia
  - Blocking action of aldosterone

- » Renal dysfunction
  - Monitor BUN & creatinine
- » Rash
- » Angioedema – luckily, it's rare, but it's scary!
  - 0.1 – 0.2% incidence
  - More common in females & African American patients
  - Elevated bradykinin, causes vasodilation
  - Can be fatal
  - Treatment of angioedema:
    - ▷ Stop the ACE-Inhibitor or ARB (no duh!)
    - ▷ Antihistamines (may not work)
    - ▷ Fresh Frozen Plasma (FFP)***
      - — Kininase II breaks down excessive bradykinin

**If cardiac catheterization/PCI is not available within 90 – 120 min, fibrinolytics may be considered:**

## Fibrinolytic Therapy

- » Tenecteplase (TNKase) - fast rapid IV bolus or
- » 5-second bolus
  - No infusion or 2nd bolus
  - Weight-based dosing no more than 50 mg
- » Activase (rtPA)
  - Bolus followed by infusion
  - Will still need to go to the Cath lab once bleeding risk is diminished

### Indications:

- » Pain < 6 hours
- » ST elevation > 1 mm in 2 or more contiguous leads

## Contraindications to fibrinolytics: (higher bleeding risk)

### Absolute:

- Active bleeding
- Intracranial hemorrhage
- Known cerebral vascular lesion
- Ischemic stroke in last 6 mos. (except acute CVA)
- Malignant intracranial neoplasm
- Suspected aortic dissection
- Closed head or facial trauma within 3 mos.
- A-V malformation

### Relative:

- Chronic, severe, poorly tolerated HTN
- SBP > 180 mm Hg or DBP > 110 mm Hg
  - lower BP prior to administration
- Ischemic CVA > 3 mos.
- Dementia
- Traumatic or prolonged CPR
- Major surgery (< 3 weeks)
- Internal bleeding (within 2 - 4 weeks)
- Pregnancy
- Active peptic ulcer disease
- Current use of anticoagulants

## Nursing Considerations post fibrinolytic administration:

- **Bleeding is the most common side effect
  - If bleeding occurs, discontinue all anticoagulants
  - Monitor PT/INR/aPTT – prolongs both
  - Monitor fibrinogen – decreased fibrinogen for up to 24°
  - Reversal – Cryoprecipitate & platelets
- Frequent neurological assessment (d/t bleeding risk)
- Avoid punctures for 6–12 hours
- Monitor urine output & BUN/creatinine
- Avoid invasive devices
- Avoid compressive devices

**Post MI Discharge: Education, education, education!**

- Medication adherence
- Minimize ETOH use
- Smoking cessation
- Exercise
- Lose weight (if applicable)
- Heart healthy diet
- Lower cholesterol & lipids
- Stress reduction

# Acute Coronary Syndrome & 12 Lead ECG

## ECG: What do the waves represent?

- P wave: Atrial depolarization
- PR interval: AV conduction time (0.12 – 0.20 sec)
- QRS: Ventricular depolarization (0.06 – 0.10 sec)
- T wave: Ventricular repolarization
- QT Interval: Time of ventricular depolarization & repolarization (0.36 - 0.44 sec)
  - QT interval is corrected because of the effect of heart rate
  - QTc = 0.4 - 0.44 sec

## Q-waves—Considered pathologic if:

- Width > 30 ms (0.04 sec)
- Depth ≥ 25% of the height of the R wave
- If present in contiguous leads, indicative of myocardial necrosis

### 12 Lead ECG Summary

| Location | ST elevation in lead: | Reciprocal changes in lead: (ST Depression) | Artery affected: | Notes: |
|---|---|---|---|---|
| Inferior | II, III, aVF | I, aVL | RCA in 65%<br>L circumflex | |
| Septal | $V_1$ - $V_2$ | II, III, aVF | LAD | |
| Anterior | $V_2$ - $V_4$ | II, III, aVF | LAD/L main | |
| Lateral | I, aVL, $V_5$ - $V_6$ | | L circumflex, LAD | |
| Posterior | Posterior leads $V_{7-9}$ | $V_{1-2}$ | RCA (90%)<br>L circumflex (10%) | Tall upright<br>R wave in $V_{1-2}$ |
| Right ventricle | $V_1$, $V_2R$ - $V_4R$ | | Proximal RCA | Right sided ECG assesses $V_2R$ - $V_4R$ |

# Types of Myocardial Infarctions

## Inferior wall MI

- Occlusion of the right coronary artery (RCA)
- Elevation in leads II, III & aVF
  - Reciprocal changes in leads I & aVL
  - Will see changes better in lead III vs. lead II

**Symptoms:**

- Bradycardia
  - Can use Atropine with caution if symptomatic
- High grade AV heart blocks—may need temporary pacer
- Second degree Type I (Wenckebach)

- » Hypotension
- » Nausea/vomiting
- » Diaphoresis
- » Monitor for signs of right ventricular infarction

## Right Ventricular Infarction

- » Associated with proximal RCA occlusion & inferior wall MI
- » May see elevation in lead $V_1$
- » If right ventricular infarction is suspected, get a right-sided ECG
  - Move precordial leads to right side of chest
  - If infarction, will see ST elevation in $V_2R - V_4R$

### Symptoms:

- » Tachycardia
- » Hypotension
- » + JVD (with clear lungs)
- » ECHO—the RV is often stunned with poor wall motion; blood backs up on the right side
- » Poor forward flow to the left side of the heart

### Treatment:

- » **IV fluids (maximize preload!)
  - Patients become preload dependent
- » Use small boluses, titrate to effect
- » + Inotrope
  - ↑ contractility
  - Dobutamine

### Avoid medications that lower preload:

- » Nitrates, morphine, beta blockers, diuretics
- » RV is often stunned and becomes preload dependent

## Anterior/Septal Wall MI

- Changes noted in $V_1$ - $V_4$
- Reciprocal changes in II, III, aVF
- Loss of R wave progression in the precordial leads ($V_1$ – $V_6$)
- Left anterior descending or left main occlusion

**Symptoms:**

- Left ventricular failure ($S_3$ heart sound)
- Shock
- Heart block
  - 2nd degree Type 2, 3rd degree
- Bundle branch block
- If new loud murmur, suspect ventricular septal rupture or papillary muscle rupture
  - Get an echocardiogram

## Conduction defects with anterior wall MI:

- Second degree type II AV block
  - Block occurs below the AV node
  - Can progress to complete heart block (CHB)
  - Constant PR interval, QRS blocked
  - If 2:1 block, can be difficult to diagnose
  - Prepare to emergently pace!
- Complete heart block (Third degree AV block)
  - No atrial impulses pass through the AV node
  - Ventricles generate their own rhythm
  - Ventricular rate is often slow—20s to 40s
  - Prepare to emergently pace!

## Lateral wall MI:

- Changes in $V_5$, $V_6$, I, aVL
- Occlusion of the left circumflex
- Can be associated with other MI locations (inferior, anterior)

## Posterior Wall MI:

- Look for tall, broad R wave (> 0.04) in $V_1$ - $V_2$ & ST depression (reciprocal change)
- Associated with inferior or lateral wall MI
- Occlusion of RCA or left circumflex
- Consider a posterior ECG
  - ST elevation in posterior leads $V_7$ - $V_9$
  - Leads follow path around the left chest wall

## Heart Blocks – Know your blocks!!!

- Here's an easy cheer to remember the different types of heart block (original author unknown)

If the R is far from the P, it means you've got a 1st degree!

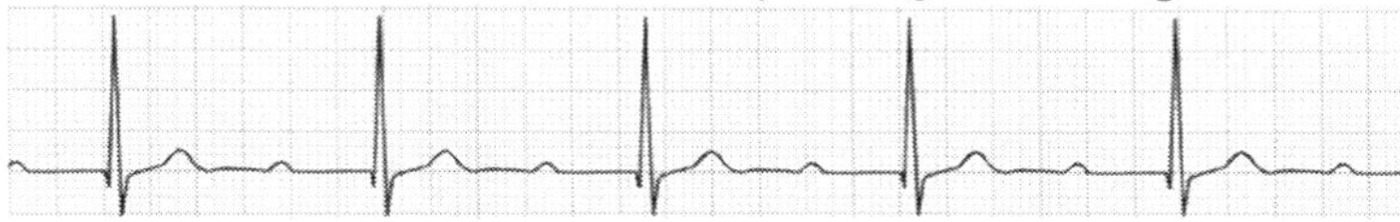

The PR interval gets longer, longer, longer, the QRS drops because it's a case of Wenckebach!

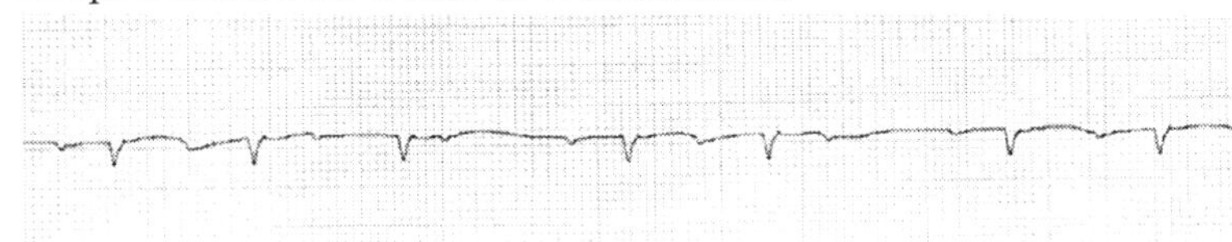

If some R's don't get through, prepare to PACE that Mobitz 2!

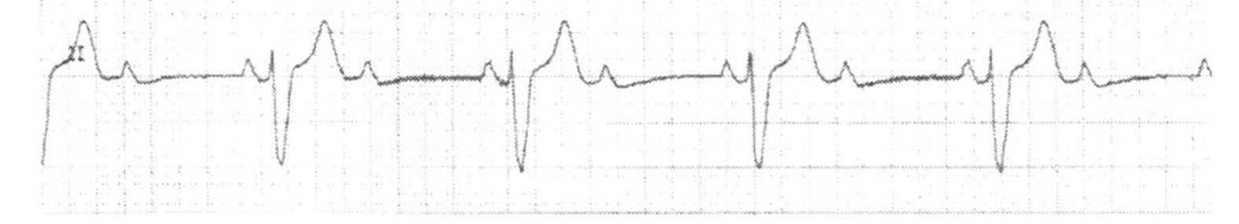

If the R's & P's don't agree, prepare to PACE that 3rd degree!!!

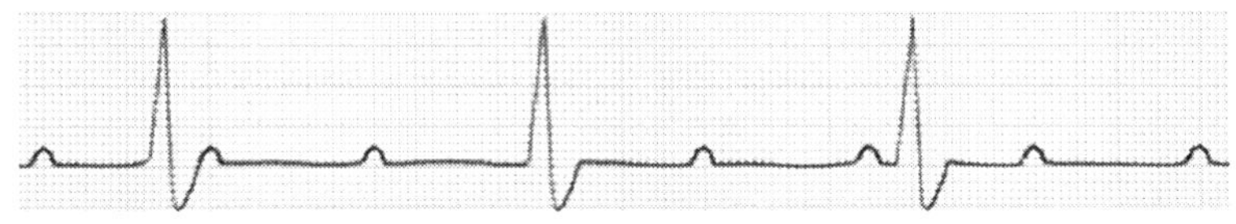

# Complications of Acute Myocardial Infarction

» A quick way to remember complications of myocardial infarctions: (Star Wars fan?!)

**D**eath
**A**rrhythmias
**R**egurgitation (valvular)
**T**amponade
**H**eart failure
**V**alve dysfunction
**A**neurysm (ventricular)
**D**ressler Syndrome
**E**mbolism
**R**upture (papillary muscle or ventricular septum)

## Pericarditis

» Inflammation of the pericardial sac

» Acute or chronic

» Chest pain—sharp, stabbing, or dull & achy

» Pain improved when sitting up, leaning forward

» Left sided radiation

» Pain worse with cough, positional changes & inspiration

» Pericardial friction rub

» Pericardial effusions

» Fever

» ECG changes observed in pericarditis:

- Diffuse ST changes; depression or elevation
- Depression of the PR interval
- Concave ST segment in limb leads
- A hint it's pericarditis & not a myocardial infarction – ST elevation in leads I & II
  - ▹ You wouldn't normally see changes in both leads in ischemia or infarction!

### Treatment:

» NSAIDs—high dose Ibuprofen

- Colchicine can also be used

» Antibiotic if bacterial, antifungal if fungus

## Papillary Muscle Rupture

» Associated w/ anterior or inferior wall MI

» Clinical signs:

- Hemodynamic instability
- New LOUD systolic murmur
- Acute MITRAL REGURG!!!
- Diagnosed by ECHO

### Treatment:

» Hemodynamic support

» Emergent surgical repair/ valve replacement

- Depends on severity

## Ventricular Septal Rupture

» At risk: anterior/septal wall MIs

» Oxygen rich blood shunts to the right side of the heart from the left

- "Left to right shunting"

### Symptoms:

» Acute SOB

» $S_3$ heart sound

» Holosystolic murmur

» Crackles

### Treatment:

» Surgery for wall repair

# Cardiogenic Shock

## Clinical signs:

- $S_3$, +JVD, pulmonary edema
- Tachycardia
- Dysrhythmias
- Signs of decreased perfusion
  - Mottling
- Decreased UOP (oliguria < 0.5 ml/kg/hr)

## Hemodynamics:

- Hypotension (MAP < 65)
- ↓ cardiac output
- ↑ afterload
- ↑ preload
- ↓ $ScvO_2$ (< 70%)
  - Drawn from a central line
  - $ScvO_2$ = Saturation of central venous oxygen

## Other diagnostics:

- ABG—Mixed respiratory & metabolic acidosis; hypoxemia
  - Lactic acidosis
- Chest x-ray: pulmonary congestion & edema
- ECHO: decreased wall motion, reduced ejection fraction
- Supportive treatment:
  - Vasopressors to support blood pressure
  - + Inotrope (i.e. Dobutamine) to improve contractility
  - Loop diuretics (as perfusion allows, ↓ preload)
  - Afterload reduction / venous vasodilators (i.e. NTG)
  - Mechanical support (i.e. IABP, Impella, ICU)

## Pulmonary Edema

- Fluid in the alveolus
- Impaired gas exchange, hypercapnia
- Hypoxemia
- Treatment: ↓ preload
  - Loop diuretics
  - Nitroglycerin
  - CPAP or BiPap

### Pharmacologic Action and Target of Vasopressors & Inotropes

| Drug | Alpha | Beta$_1$ | Beta$_2$ |
|---|---|---|---|
| Phenylephrine | ++++ | - | - |
| Norepinephrine | ++++ | ++ | - |
| Dopamine | ++<br>< 5mcg/kg/min | ++++<br>< 10 mcg/kg/min | + |
| | +++<br>> 10mcg/kg/min | | |
| Dobutamine | + | ++++ | ++ |

**Note: In the AACN blueprint, it states you need to know Dopamine, Dobutamine and Nitroglycerin**

### Adrenergic receptors:

- Alpha—located in blood vessels
- Beta$_1$— located on the heart
- Beta$_2$— located in the bronchial & vascular smooth muscle

## **Vasopressors** (Used to increase blood pressure):

### Dopamine (Inotropin)

- Effect: ↑HR, ↑BP
- Classified as a catecholamine
- Acts on the sympathetic nervous system (SNS)
- Positive inotropic effects

- Monitor closely for extravasation
- Stimulates $Beta_1$ & some $Beta_2$, alpha
- Watch out for tachy arrhythmias & ventricular ectopy

**Dosing:**

- 0.5 - 3 mcg/kg/min—dopaminergic receptors
  - may see ↑ in BP
- 3 - 10 mcg/kg/min—beta effects (+ inotrope)
  - ↑ C.O.
- > 10 mcg/kg/min—alpha effects (vasoconstriction)
  - ↑ BP
- Max. 20 mcg/kg/min

## Norepinephrine (Levophed)

- Effect: ↑ BP
- Alpha & $Beta_1$
- Adverse effects: bradycardia, dysrhythmias, HTN, renal artery vasoconstriction
- Dosing: 0.5 – 30 mcg/min—titrate to effect
- Monitor closely for extravasation
- Vasopressor of choice in sepsis guidelines
  - That's why I kept it in this study guide for you!

## Phenylephrine (Neo-Synephrine)

- Effect: ↑ BP
- Pure alpha
- Adverse effects: reflexive bradycardia, dysrhythmias, HTN, chest pain
- Dosing: 2 - 10 mcg/kg/min
- Titrate to effect/BP parameters established
- Monitor closely for extravasation

## Positive Inotropes (Used to improve cardiac output & contractility):

### Dobutamine (Dobutrex)

- » Effect: ↑ C.O., ↑ UOP
- » Stimulates beta receptors, $Beta_1$ (some alpha)
- » Also used in cardiac surgery & septic shock
- » Dosing: 2 – 20 mcg/kg/min IV (up to 40 mcg/kg/min)
- » Onset 1 - 2 minutes, up to 10 min.
- » Plasma half-life 2 min.
- » Monitor for: tachycardia, hypotension, hypertension, ectopy, hypokalemia

### Milrinone (Primacor)

- » Effect ↑ C.O., ↓ preload & ↓ afterload, no change in HR
- » Phosphodiesterase (PDE) inhibitor
- » Vasodilatory effects—watch BP!
- » Dosing: Bolus 50 mcg/kg over 10 min.
  - Maintenance: 0.375 – 0.75 mcg/kg/min
  - FYI—I've rarely seen a bolus given
- » Long half-life!!!!
  - ~ 2½ hours

# Cardiac Surgery

## Coronary Artery Bypass Graft (CABG)

- » Artery harvested from:
  - Saphenous vein (leg)
  - Internal mammary
  - Radial artery
    - ▹ Can spasm
    - ▹ Use NTG &/or CCB

### Post-op considerations:

- » Longer cardiopulmonary bypass time =
  - Increased risk of bleeding
  - Increased risk of stroke & neurologic injury

**Monitor:**

- BP (↑ BP = risk for bleeding)
- Pain
- Electrolyte imbalances
- Bleeding
- Post-op ischemia
- Dysrhythmias/blocks
  - Atrial fibrillation
- Fluid overload
- **Ateletasis**
  - Cough & deep breath!
  - Incentive spirometer

**Teaching after surgery:**

- Sternal precautions
- Cough & deep breath
- Signs of infection
- Weight gain
- Heart healthy diet
  - Low sodium
- ↑ Activity/exercise
- Smoking cessation
- Medication adherence
- DVT prophylaxis

## Cardiac Tamponade

- Compression of the heart due to fluid or blood accumulation within the pericardium
- The pericardial space normally contains 20 – 50 ml of pericardial fluid
- Clinical signs/symptoms of cardiac tamponade:
  - **Beck's Triad**:
    - Elevated CVP w/JVD
    - Hypotension
    - Muffled heart sounds
  - Sudden drop in chest tube output
  - Narrow pulse pressure (SBP – DBP = PP)
    - Normal PP = 40 mm Hg
  - Tachycardia
  - Electrical alternans
    - Alternating beat variation of amplitude on ECG
  - Pulsus paradoxus
    - > 10 mm Hg drop in BP during inspiration
  - Wide mediastinum on chest xray
  - Pulseless Electrical Activity (PEA)

**Treatment of cardiac tamponade:**

- Pericardiocentesis if medical cause
  - Risk: Laceration of coronary artery
- Median re-sternotomy if surgical bleeding
- Goal: Locate & control source of bleeding

# Arrythmias

## Atrial fibrillation/atrial flutter

**General risk factors for developing afib/aflutter:**

- CABG
- Valvular disease
- MI
- Obesity
- Atherosclerosis
- Rheumatic heart disease
- Lung disease

**Rates can vary:**

- > 100 bpm "Rapid ventricular response"
- Lose atrial kick
- ↓ in C.O. by up to 20 - 25%

## Management of afib/aflutter:

**Rate control vs. conversion**

- Synchronized cardioversion if new (vs. chronic) & UNSTABLE!
- Digoxin
- Beta blockers (esmolol, metoprolol)
  - Use cautiously in patients with reduced EF
  - Has negative inotropic effects

- Calcium channel blockers (diltiazem)
  - Use cautiously in patients with reduced EF
  - Has negative inotropic effects
- Amiodarone—safer to use with reduced ejection fraction
- Anticoagulation if sustained in afib

### Supraventricular Tachycardia (SVT)

- Stable vs. unstable (unstable = cardioversion)
- If stable, remember this acronym:
- **V**agal maneuvers
- **A**denosine 6 mg IV - **Rapid**!!!
  - Repeat 12 mg x 2, every 1 – 2 min
  - Depresses AV node conduction
  - Instruct patient prior to administration – they may feel breathless
- **D**iltiazem IV

# Heart Failure

## 2 types:

### Heart Failure with preserved EF (HFpEF)

- **Diastolic Heart Failure**
- Ejection Fraction (EF) ≥ 50%
- Borderline EF 41 – 49%
- Usually history of hypertension
- Stiff non-compliant ventricle and left ventricular hypertrophy (LVH)
- Treatment focuses on controlling BP

### Heart Failure with reduced EF (HFrEF)

- **Systolic Heart Failure**
- Ejection Fraction ≤ 40%
- aka: "congestive heart failure"
- Acute decompensated HF
- Know HFrEF well for the exam!

## Ventricular failure—left vs. right side

### Left sided failure—blood backs up to the lungs

- ↓ CO/CI
- Tachypnea
- Tachycardia
- $S_3$ heart sound
- Mitral regurgitation
- Crackles
- Cough, frothy sputum
- ↑ Pulmonary arterial pressures
- ↑ Preload, ↑ afterload
- Displaced point of maximal impulse (PMI)

### Right sided failure—blood backs up to the venous periphery

- JVD
- Hepatojugular reflux
- Peripheral edema
- Hepatomegaly
- Anorexia, N/V
- Ascites
- Tricuspid regurgitation
- ↑ Preload (↑ CVP)
- ↑ Liver enzymes

## Assessment in heart failure:

### Measuring JVD

- Supine position, HOB 30°
- Turn head slightly to left—note: the right jugular is aligned directly with the right atrium
- Observe for pulsations
- Note highest point
- Measure distance between the pulsation & sternal angle
- 4 cm above sternal angle is normal

### PMI (Point of maximum impulse)

- Normally palpated at the 5th ICS, MCL

**Causes of PMI shifting:**

- Left ventricular hypertrophy
- Heart failure
- Right pneumothorax
- Right pleural effusion

## Heart failure (HFrEF)

### HFrEF - Reduced EF Systolic Heart Failure

- Damage to myofibrils
- Results in ↑ preload & ↑ afterload
- Elevated BNP Levels
  - Hormone secreted by ventricles in response to stretch

### General medical management

**All aimed at blocking the sympathetic nervous system (SNS), renin angiotensin aldosterone system (RAAS), Aldosterone & Neprilysin**
***The end of this chapter has additional info on meds!***

- ACE inhibitor <u>OR</u> angiotensin receptor blocker (ARB) <u>OR</u>
- Angiotensin Receptor Blocker/ Neprilysin Inhibitor (ARNI)
  - Entresto
- Beta-blocker <u>OR</u> alpha/ beta blocker
  - Bisoprolol
  - Metoprolol succinate
  - Carvedilol
- Aldosterone antagonist (i.e. spironolactone)
- Hydralazine (afterload reducer) + isosorbide dinitrate (preload reducer)
- Vasodilators (nitrates)
- Diuretics (usually loop)
- Cardiac glycosides (i.e. digoxin)

## Entresto™ (sacubitril/valsartan) - FYI

- Class: ARB/Neprilysin inhibitor (ARNI)
- Indicated to reduce the risk of cardiovascular death & hospitalization for heart failure (HF) in patients with chronic heart failure (CHF) (NYHA class II-IV) & reduced ejection fraction
- Recommended starting dose: 49 mg/51 mg PO BID
  - Target maintenance dose:
  - After 2 - 4 weeks, double the dose to the target maintenance dose of 97 mg/103 mg PO BID as tolerated
- 20% mortality reduction compared to Enalapril
- Usually used as a 2nd line agent

## Acute decompensated heart failure

- Dobutamine or Milrinone infusions
  - Improve contractility, ↓ afterload
- Diuretics
  - Remove fluid
  - ↓ preload
- Nitroglycerin
  - ↓ preload
  - Some effect to ↓ afterload
- Nesiritide (Natrecor)
  - Sometimes used in acute decompensated HF without cardiogenic shock
  - Potent vasodilator
  - Dilates arteries to ↓ preload & afterload, ↑ C.O.
  - Inhibits the renin-angiotensin-aldosterone system
  - Dosing: bolus 2 mcg/kg over 1 minute
    - Maintenance: 0.01 mcg/kg/min
    - Short half-life (~18 minutes)
  - Monitor for hypotension

## Long term heart failure options

- » Biventricular pacing if the patient has a BBB
- » Cardiac assist devices (LVAD, RVAD or BiVAD)
- » Cardiac transplant
- » + Inotropes (i.e. Dobutamine or Milrinone)
  - Can be used palliative

### Ventricular Assist Device (VADS)

- » Left (LVAD), right (RVAD) or both (BiVAD)

#### Short term

- » Bridge to transplant

#### Long term

- » Destination therapy LVAD

## Cardiac transplantation

- » Vagal nerve is severed
- » Atropine will not work if bradycardic—need to pace!
- » Immunosuppression to prevent rejection
- » Prevent infection!

## Cardiac Resynchronization Therapy

- » Biventricular Pacemaker
- » Used in heart failure when patient has low EF & BBB
  - Indicated for EF < 35% with a QRS duration > 0.12 sec
- » Bi-ventricular pacing results in shortened QRS duration and better ventricular synchrony

**Benefits:**

- Synchronized ventricular contraction
- Increased EF/C.O.
- Symptom improvement
- Complement medical therapy
- Improve quality of life
- Give hope to those who are suffering with moderate to severe heart failure
- No mortality benefits shown

## Heart Failure Diagnostics

- 12 Lead ECG—Assess for ischemia, BBB
- Chest radiograph—assess for fluid overload, heart enlargement
- ECHO
- Trans-Esophageal ECHO (TEE)—assess heart function, wall motion and presence of thrombus
- Angiogram indicated if ischemic

### Heart Failure Discharge Education

- Medication adherence
- Activity
- Daily weight
- Sodium restricted diet
    - Strict $Na^+$ & fluid restriction debatable; fluid restrict if hyponatremic, $Na^+$ restrict if pulmonary congestion
    - $Na^+$ is a major nemesis in heart failure!
- Smoking (and other health habits—quit smoking, limit alcohol intake, lose weight)
- Prevent infection—flu & pneumococcal vaccines

## Hypertrophic Obstructive Cardiomyopathy (HOCM)

### Physiologic changes:

- » Thickened interventricular septum
- » Diastolic dysfunction and left ventricular hypertrophy (LVH)
- » Decreased compliance & aortic outflow obstruction
- » Assessment: $S_4$, murmur, displaced PMI
- » May present with sudden cardiac death
- » Treatment: beta blocker &/ or calcium channel blockers
- » Goal—slow the heart rate to prolong diastole & filling time!
- » Avoid inotropes!!! (i.e. Digoxin/Dobutamine)
- » Reduce septum:
  - Percutaneous transluminal septal myocardial ablation (PTSMA)
  - Alcohol ablation of septum
  - Septal Myomectomy—removing septal muscle that is contributing to aortic outflow obstruction
- » Implantable Cardioverter Defibrillator (ICD)— treat sudden cardiac death & ventricular arrhythmias

## Takotsubo Cardiomyopathy

- » Also called “Broken Heart Syndrome” or “Stress Induced Cardiomyopathy”
- » Result of severe emotional or physical stress
- » Possibly the result of a surge in stress hormones (i.e. adrenalin)
- » Weakening & ballooning of the left ventricle
- » Reversible, happens almost exclusively in women—~90%
- » Often resolves within one month

### Symptoms:

- » Chest pain
- » SOB
- » Can see ST elevations on the 12 Lead ECG
- » Coronary cath is often clean

### Treatment:

- Standard heart failure meds—ACE inhibitor or ARB, beta blocker, loop diuretics, aldosterone antagonists (spironolactone)

# Murmurs & Valve Dysfunction

## Murmurs—2 causes:

### StenOsis:

- Forward flow of blood through stenotic open valves

### Insufficiency/Regurgitation:

- Backward flow through incompetently closed valves
- Murmurs are high pitched except murmurs of stenosis

### Systolic murmurs

- Pulmonary & aortic stenOsis are systolic murmurs...
  - Murmurs of stenOsis are auscultated when valves are Open!
  - The pulmonic & aortic valves are Open during systole
  - Therefore, they are systolic murmurs!
- Tricuspid & mitral regurg/insufficiency are systolic murmurs...
  - Murmurs of insufficiency are auscultated when valves are closed!
  - The tricuspid & mitral valves are closed during systole
  - Therefore, they are systolic murmurs!
- Auscultate on and between $S_1$ and $S_2$ (during systole)
- $S_1$ - murmur - $S_2$

### Diastolic murmurs

» Tricuspid & mitral stenOsis are diastolic murmurs...

- Murmurs of stenOsis are auscultated when valves are Open!
- The tricuspid & mitral valves are Open during diastole
- Therefore, they are diastolic murmurs!

» Pulmonary & aortic regurgitation/insufficiency are diastolic murmurs...

- Murmurs of insufficiency are auscultated when valves are closed!
- The pulmonic & aortic valves are closed during diastole
- Therefore, they are diastolic murmurs

» Auscultate after $S_2$ (during diastole)

» $S_1$ - $S_2$ - murmur

| Type of murmur | Systolic or Diastolic? | Location |
|---|---|---|
| Mitral/Tricuspid Stenosis | Diastolic | 5th ICS, MCL (M) |
| Mitral/Tricuspid Regurg | Systolic | 5th ICS, MCL (M) |
| Aortic/Pulmonic Stenosis | Systolic | 2nd ICS, RSB (A) |
| Aortic/Pulmonic Regurg | Diastolic | 2nd ICS, RSB (A) |

# Valvular Dysfunction

## Mitral Insufficiency/Regurgitation

» Systolic murmur

### Causes:

» MI

» Ruptured chordae tendineae

» Severe left heart failure

» Left ventricular hypertrophy

- Cardiomyopathy
- Mitral valve prolapse
- Rheumatic Heart Disease
- Myxomatous degeneration
- Endocarditis

**Symptoms:**

- **SYSTOLIC murmur**
- Orthopnea/dyspnea
- Fatigue
- Angina
- Increased left atrial pressure
- Right heart failure
- Prone to atrial fibrillation d/t left atrial enlargement
- Left heart failure

**Treatment:**

- Medical management targeted to reduce preload & afterload
- Mitral valve clip (if a candidate)
  - MitraClip®
- Mitral valve replacement

## Mitral Stenosis

- Auscultate when the mitral valve is OPEN
- Diastolic murmur

**Signs & Symptoms:**

- Pinkish cheeks
- Pulmonary edema
- Prone to afib (due to atrial enlargement)
- Increased right heart pressures
- Pulmonary hypertension

### Treatment:

- Medical management
  - Aimed at reducing preload & afterload
- Valve repair
  - Commissurotomy
- Surgical replacement
- Balloon Valvuloplasty
  - ↑ diameter/opening of valve

### Mitral valve dysfunction:

**Atrial enlargement is often seen with mitral valve dysfunction**
**This makes patients prone to atrial fibrillation**
**What you might see on the 12 Lead ECG:**

- Right atrial enlargement:
  - P wave amplitude > 2.5 mm in II and/or > 1.5 mm in V1
  - QR, Qr, qR, or qRs morphology in lead V1 (without CAD)
- Left atrial enlargement:
  - P wave duration ≥ 0.12 sec (usually lead II)
  - Notched P wave in limb leads with the inter-peak duration ≥ 0.04 sec
- Bi-atrial enlargement:
  - Features of both RAE & LAE in same ECG
  - P wave in lead II > 2.5 mm tall & ≥ 0.12 in duration

## Aortic Insufficiency/Regurgitation

- Diastolic murmur
- Results in a backflow of blood & reduced diastolic pressure
- Over time, leads to left ventricular hypertrophy

### Causes:

- Chronic hypertension
- Rheumatic Heart Disease
- Endocarditis
- Marfan's Syndrome
- Idiopathic—means we don't know why!

### Symptoms:

- DeMusset sign—head bobbing
- Brisk carotid upstroke
- Wide pulse pressure
  - > 40 mm Hg
  - High systolic BP; low diastolic BP
- "Water-hammer" pulse—rapid upstroke & down stroke with a shortened peak

## Aortic Stenosis

- Auscultate when the aortic valve is OPEN
- Systolic murmur
- Systolic ejection is impeded
- LV hypertrophy due to ↑ resistance
- Pressure gradient between LV & aorta
  - Pressure higher in LV
- 50%, 2-year mortality if HF develops

### Symptoms:

- Heart failure
- Activity intolerance
- SOB
- Chronic ↑ afterload due to narrow stenotic valve

### Treatment:

- Surgical valve replacement
- Trans-Catheter Aortic Valve Replacement (TAVR)
- Post TAVR replacement, monitor for stroke & bradycardia or heart block
  - May need long term pacemaker
  - Monitor insertion site for bleeding or hematoma

## Valvular diagnosis

» Echocardiogram (gold standard)

» Cardiac catheterization (may see ↓CO, ↑preload & ↑atrial pressure)

» 12 lead ECG: left atrial & ventricular hypertrophy

» Chest x-ray: left atrial & ventricular enlargement, pulmonary venous congestion

### Treatment:

» Treat heart failure if present:
- ACE inhibitor or ARB
  - ▹ Blunt RAAS
- Beta blocker
  - ▹ Blunt the SNS
- Diuretics
- Afterload reduction (hydralazine), ACE-Inhibitor or ARB

» Valve repair/replacement

# Acute Inflammatory Diseases

**"itis" = inflammation**

**Overview of cardiac inflammatory diseases:**

**MYOcarditis**
- Inflammation of the muscle
- Chest pain, failure, arrythmias
- Viral, toxins, infiltrates

**PERIcarditis**
- Inflammation of sac surrounding the heart
- Sharp pain, ST↑ on ECG, pericardial rub
- May be viral cause
- Use anti-inflammatory medications

**ENDOcarditis**
- Inflammation of the inner lining of the heart
- Murmur, night sweats, fever
- IV drug use, bad teeth
- Antibiotics

## Myocarditis

- Focal or diffuse inflammation of the myocardium
- Viral or bacterial infection

### Clinical signs:

- Fever, chest pain, heart failure, dysrhythmias, sudden cardiac death
- May be accompanied by pericarditis

### Treatment:

- Antibiotics (if bacterial)
- NSAIDs
- Diuretics
- + inotropes
  - Improve contractility
- ACE inhibitor
  - ↓ afterload

## Pericarditis

- Inflammation of the pericardial sac
- Constrictive: fibrous deposits on the pericardium
- Restrictive: effusions into the pericardial sac

### Causes:

- Acute MI, post-CABG, connective tissue disease, infection
  - 10 - 15% develop this 2 - 7 days after AMI
- Dressler's syndrome:
  - 2 - 12 weeks after MI
  - Caused from an autoimmune response or viral infection

## Symptoms:

- Retrosternal PLEURITIC chest pain
- Pain is worse:
  - On inspiration (deep breath)
  - Supine position
  - With activity
  - Pain is relieved by leaning forward
- Pericardial friction rub
- Tachycardia
- Tachypnea
- Fever

## ECG findings with pericarditis:

- Concave diffuse ST segment elevation
  - Especially precordial leads
- Tall peaked T waves in numerous leads
  - Except lead aVR
- Down-sloping TP segment
  - Called Spodick's sign
- Depressed PR interval

## Treatment:

- Time
- Prevent/relieve symptoms (positioning)
  - Leaning forward pulls heart away from diaphragmatic pleurae of lungs
- NSAIDs
- Corticosteroids if NSAIDs are ineffective
- If infective in nature: antibiotic, antiviral – whatever is appropriate
- Monitor for **complications** of pericarditis:
  - Pleural effusion
  - Constrictive pericarditis
  - Cardiac tamponade
- Chronic pericarditis: partial pericardiectomy
  - Window created allowing fluids to drain into pleural space
- Constrictive pericarditis: total pericardiectomy

## Endocarditis

- Infection of the endocardium or valve
- Damaged leaflets

### Causes:

- Trauma
- Bacteria

### At risk:

- Cardiac surgery
- Rheumatic heart disease
- Dental procedures
- IV drug abuse (especially tricuspid & pulmonic valve)

### Symptoms:

- Stabbing, sharp pain
  - Worse on inspiration
  - May radiate to neck, shoulders, back and arms
- SOB, cough
- JVD
- Pulsus paradoxus
- Pericardial friction rub
- ST elevations
- Narrow pulse pressure
- Elevated WBC, ESR
- Monitor for neurologic impairment
  - Vegetation embolism leading to stroke

### Endocarditis common organisms:

- Streptococcus
- Staphylococcus
- Gram negative bacilli
- Fungus (i.e. candida)
- Administer appropriate antibiotics

## Assessment findings with inflammatory diseases:

### Pulsus paradoxus

- ↓ in systolic pressure during inspiration; > 10 mm Hg
- Caused by cardiac tamponade, pleural effusion, pericarditis or dehydration

### Pulsus alternans

- Finding on arterial waveform showing alternating strong and weak beats
- Indicative of left ventricular systolic impairment

### Pericardial Rubs

- Scratching, grating, squeaking leather quality
- Left lower sternal border, leaning forward or lying supine in deep expiration
- High frequency
- 3 sounds are present
  - One systolic—occurs anywhere in systole
  - Two diastolic—occurs w/ ventricular stretch at early and late diastole
- Auscultated in MI, pericarditis, autoimmune, trauma, s/p cardiac surgery, autoimmune diseases

## Overall "itis" treatment goals:

- Prevent/relieve symptoms
- NSAIDs (ASA or indomethacin)
- Treat infection
- Corticosteroids

# Conduction issues

## Tachycardias

- Tachycardia—Narrow complex (SVT)
  - Stable vs. unstable
  - Unstable: Prepare for cardioversion!
  - Stable? Narrow & regular complex?
    - **V**agal maneuvers
    - **A**denosine
      - Dosed: 6 mg, 12 mg, 12 mg by RAPID IVP
      - Used in SVT
      - Depresses AV node conduction
      - Instruct patient prior to administration
    - **D**iltiazem IV
- Tachycardia—Wide complex
  - QRS > 0.12 sec; consult an expert
  - Amiodarone 150 mg IV over 10 min.
  - Can also use Lidocaine for monomorphic wide complex tachycardia
  - Since 2010 AHA ACLS guidelines:
    - Adenosine 6 mg IV, may repeat

## Long QT syndrome (LQTS)

- Delayed repolarization can cause Torsade de Pointes (polymorphic ventricular tachycardia)
- Present with fainting or sudden cardiac death
- Prolonged QT, QTc > 450 ms
- Can also result from malnutrition due to $K^+$ & $Mg^{++}$ deficiencies

### Treatment:

- Genetic testing
- Electrolyte supplements
- Beta blockers
- Antidysrhythmic based on cause of LQTS
- Implantable cardioverter defibrillator (ICD)

## Brugada Syndrome

» Genetic cause of sudden cardiac death

» Sodium channelopathy

### Symptoms:

» Fainting, irregular heart beats

» Coved or saddle-back ST elevations in leads $V_1 - V_3$

» Often have a right BBB

» Long PR interval

» May have short QT interval; < 360 ms

» Structural right ventricle pathology

### Treatment:

» Implantable cardioverter defibrillator (ICD)

» Possibly quinidine

## Antidysrhythmic Medications:

| Class | Medication | Effect | Uses |
|---|---|---|---|
| IA | Quinidine (Cardioquin)*<br>Procainamide (Pronestyl)* | Prolongs repolarization | Atrial or ventricular dysrhythmia monitor QTc interval - will prolong |
| IB | Lidocaine (Xylocaine)*<br>Tocainamide (Tonocard)<br>Mexiletin (Mexitil) | Shortens action potential duration | Ventricular dysrhythmias |
| IC | Flecainamide (Tambocor)<br>Propafenone (Rhythmol) | Blocks $Na^+$ channels | Ventricular dysrhythmias |
| II | Propanolol (Inderal)<br>Esmolol (Brevibloc)* | Decreases HR & SA node automaticity Beta blocker | Atrial dysrhythmias & SVT |

| Class | Medication | Effect | Uses |
|---|---|---|---|
| III | Amiodarone (Cordarone)** <br> Bretylium (Bretylol) <br> Sotalol (Betapace) | Blocks $K^+$ channels, slows conduction | Atrial & ventricular dysrhythmias |
| IV | Verapamil (Calan)* <br> Diltiazem (Cardizem)* | Calcium channel antagonist | Atrial tachycardia & atrial flutter |
| Other | Digoxin (Lanoxin)* <br> Adenosine (Adenocard)* | Slows AV node conduction, depresses SA node | Atrial fibrilation, atrial flutter & SVT |

# Digoxin/Lanoxin

- Loading dose: 1.0 - 1.5 mg over 24 hours
  - Average dose is 0.125 - 0.25 mg daily
- Therapeutic range 0.5 - 2.0
  - Check level 6 - 8 hours after dose
- Digoxin can cause almost any arrhythmia
- Digoxin effects & uses:
  - Increases myocardial contractility
  - Slows conduction of impulse through the AV node
  - Used to control ventricular rate in atrial fibrillation or atrial flutter
    - May be best suited for use in patients with heart failure & atrial fibrillation
  - Does not reduce mortality, but may be helpful for symptom control
  - Hypokalemia ↑ risk of Dig toxicity
- Signs of Digoxin toxicity:
  - Bradycardia
  - Prolonged PR interval – 1st degree AV conduction delay
  - Prolonged QT interval
  - Vision changes
  - Nausea/vomiting
  - Dizziness
- Look for meds that ↑ or ↓ effects of digoxin:
  - Amiodarone
    - Increases Dig level
    - Usually ↓ dose by 1/2 when amiodarone is started

- PPIs
  - Increases Dig level
- Antacids
  - Decreases bioavailability of Dig

## Wolfe-Parkinson-White (WPW)

» Pre-excitation

» Abnormal conduction pathway between the atria & ventricles

» Accessory pathways conduct faster than the AV node

» Short PR interval < 0.12 sec

» Delta wave—slurred upstroke in the QRS

### Treatment:

» Ablation of the accessory pathway

» Antiarrhythmic medications slow conduction

- Beta blockers often used

» Avoid digoxin, calcium channel blockers & Adenosine

» Can cardiovert in the short term if unstable

## Pacemaker Review

» Permanent or temporary

» Indications: symptomatic bradycardia, 2nd degree AV block (Mobitz II), third degree AV block (complete heart block)

» Patients admitted with "Syncope" will require f/u electrophysiology study

» Transcutaneous, transvenous, epicardial are ways to temporary pace a patient

- Transvenous pacing usually done in the ICU

## Temporary—Transcutaneous Pacing

» Pad placement: Anterior–posterior or anterior–lateral

» Settings include:

- Mode of pacing (Demand)
- Pacing rate (Usually 60 – 80)
- Energy (mA)

» Demand (synchronous) mode

- Preferred mode of pacing
- Mode is usually VVI

» Fixed (asynchronous) mode

- Avoid as a pacing mode
- Will pace regardless of patient's intrinsic rhythm
- Potential issue: R on T, causing lethal dysrhythmias
- Can be dangerous & cause R on T arrythmias

» More energy required vs. transvenous

- Start @ 50 mA & ↑ until capture
- Pacing spike immediately follwed by a wide QRS
- Need to pace through skin, bone, muscle

## Pacing Codes

### Pacemaker codes: Example—VVI, AAI, DDD

» First letter: Chamber paced (A, V or D)

» Second letter: Chamber sensed (A, V or D)

» Third letter: Response to sensing

- I—Inhibits pacing if QRS is sensed, demand
- D—Inhibits pacing in both chambers
- O—None
- Typically, we want the response to pacing set in either I or D
- This means if the patient has their own intrinsic rhythm, the pacemaker will sense it and not compete with the patient

### Examples:

- VVI – V: ventricle is paced, V: ventricle is sensed, I: pacing will be inhibited if the pacemaker senses intrinsic conduction
- DDD – D: atria & ventricle are paced, D: atria & ventricle are sensed, D: pacing will be inhibited if the pacemaker senses intrinsic conduction

## Failure to capture:

- Electrical stimulus delivered (pacing spike), but no electrical capture (wide QRS)

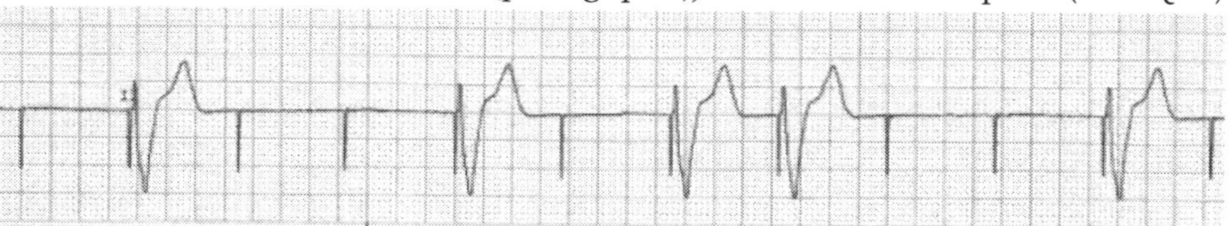

### Causes:

- Improper position of wire or pads
- Low voltage
- Battery failure
- Inadequate/loose connection
- Fibrosis of catheter tip
  - Transvenous

### Troubleshooting:

- Check connections
- ↑ mA (energy)
- Assess pH, electrolyte imbalances, ischemia & drug toxicity
  - May require much higher mA to capture

## Failure to pace:

- Pacing stimulus is not delivered to the myocardium

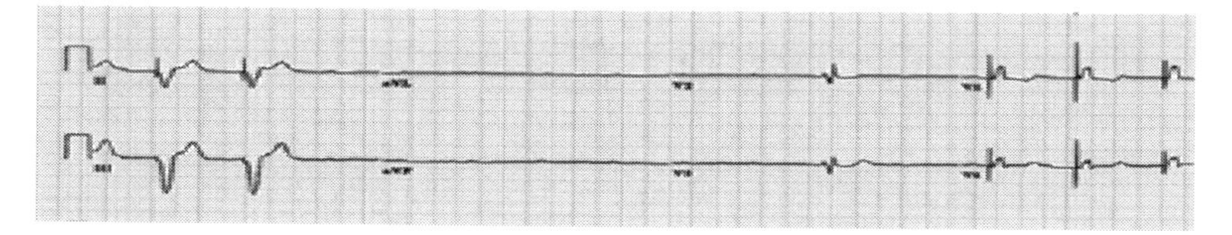

### Causes:

- Battery failure
- Lead dislodgement
- Loose connections
- Improper settings

### Troubleshooting:

- Assess leads & connections
- Assess thresholds
- Assess labs
- Change battery
- Prepare for transcutaneous pacing (TCP)

## Failure to sense:

- Under-sensing: the pacemaker does not recognize intrinsic beats
  - Dangerous, because patient can experience R on T arrhythmia
- Over-sensing: the pacemaker thinks that either P waves or T waves are ventricular depolarization & does not pace

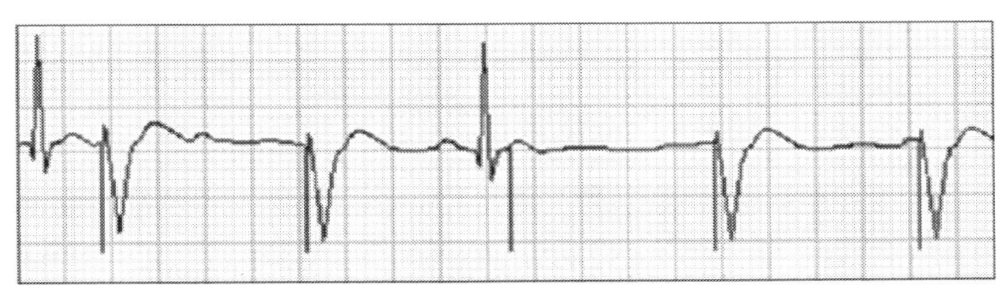

This is an example of under-sensing. The pacemaker didn't "see" or sense the R wave & pacing spike was delivered on the T wave.

### Causes:

- Improper sensitivity settings
- Position of the lead

### Troubleshooting:

- Assess sensitivity threshold
- For PPM, interrogation needs to be performed

### Magnet Operation with Permanent Pacemakers & ICDs

- A magnet placed over a pacemaker causes asynchronous pacing at a designated "magnet" rate
  - Does NOT turn off the pacemaker...a common misconception!!!
- Over an ICD, a magnet inhibits defibrillation
- A magnet might be used in surgery if cautery is used or if a defibrillator is mis-firing
- Terminates pacemaker mediated tachycardia

## Cardiac Arrest & Resuscitation

- Early CPR with **minimal** interruptions
- Compressions of good quality
  - 100 - 120/minute
  - 2 - 2.4 inch depth
- Early defibrillation
  - Minimize pauses
  - Escalate energy
- Avoid excessive ventilation
  - 10 breaths/min or 30:2
- Figure out cause
  - 5 H's, 5 T's

### Types of arrest & treatment strategies:

- Ventricular Fibrillation
  - **S**hock (if readily available); Repeat Q 2 min.
  - **C**PR for 2 min
  - **R**hythm check - shock if warranted
  - **E**pi 1 mg IV/IO Q 3 - 5 min
  - **A**miodarone 300 mg IV/IO; repeat bolus 150 mg IV/IO if still in VF/VT
  - **M**edications (other): Lidocaine 1.0 - 1.5 mg/kg IV/IO
- Torsades de pointes
  - "Polymorphic" ventricular tacycardia
  - Shift in axis
  - Caused by hypomagnesemia, prolonged QT, multiple medications
  - Also caused by methadone & some quinolones
    - Cause prolonged QT interval
  - Treatment: magnesium sulfate 1 - 2 grams IV/IO (diluted)
  - Magnesium antagonist: calcium chloride

- PEA (pulseless electrical activity)
  - **P**ump: Start compressions
  - **E**pinephrine 1 mg IV/ IO Q 3 - 5 min
  - **A**ssess causes
- Asystole
  - No cardiac output or electrical activity
  - **P**ump (Same as PEA)
  - **E**pinephrine 1 mg IV/ IO Q 3 - 5 min
  - **A**ssess differential diagnosis
  - Consider termination if Capnography < 10 mm Hg after 20 min
- Causes:
  - **5 H's:**
    - Hypovolemia
    - Hypoxia
    - Hypo/Hyperkalemia
    - H+ ion (acidosis)
    - Hypothermia
  - **5 T's:**
    - Thrombus:
      - MI
      - PE
    - Tension pneumothorax
    - Tamponade
    - Toxicology (drug OD)
- Capnography during resuscitation
  - Normal $PEtCO_2$ 35 - 45 mm Hg
  - Minimum goal > 10 mm Hg
  - Used as a marker of perfusion & chest compression quality
  - If less than 10, improve quality of compressions
  - If rapid ↑ in $PEtCO_2$, may be a sign of ROSC
  - If consistently < 10 mm Hg in the setting of adequate compressions, discuss termination of resuscitation efforts

## Post-arrest care

- Optimize hemodynamics
  - Avoid hypotension
  - Avoid hypoxemia or hyperoxemia
- Reperfusion
  - Obtain 12 Lead ECG
  - Does the patient need to go to the Cath lab?
- Targeted Temperature Management (TTM)
  - 32 - 36°C for 24 hours
  - Recommended for all rhythms & in-hospital arrest
    - Reason: neuro protection
  - Avoid fever for at least 48° after TTM protocol is complete
  - See Neurology section for more info

# Cardiac Trauma

## Penetrating trauma, common injury to:

- » Chambers of the heart
- » Right ventricle
- » Pericardium
- » Great vessels/coronary arteries
- » Risk of infection
- » Surgical emergency

## Blunt trauma, common causes:

- » MVC/steering wheel to chest
- » Direct blow to chest
- » Fall
- » Stunned or contused myocardium
- » Ventricular rupture
- » Acceleration/deceleration injury: vessel damage
- » Direct transfer mechanics

## Blunt Cardiac Injury

- » Formerly called "cardiac contusion"
- » Right atrium & ventricle most at risk

### Monitor for:

- » Dysrhythmias
- » Heart block/right BBB

### Medical management:

- » Prevent complications
- » Antidysrhythmics
- » Heart failure
- » Temporary pacing

### Diagnosis:

» ECHO, 12 Lead ECG, CXR, CT Scan, MRI, Trans Esophageal Echo (TEE)

» Cardiac enzymes

» Other labs: Coags, electrolytes, CBC

# Hypertension

| Category | SBP | | DBP |
|---|---|---|---|
| Normal | < 120 | and | < 80 |
| Elevated | 120 - 129 | and | < 80 |
| Stage 1 HTN | 130 - 139 | or | 80-89 |
| Stage 2 HTN | ≥ 140 | or | ≥ 90 |
| Hypertensive Crisis | > 180 | and/or | > 120 |

Source: 2017 AHA Hypertension Guidelines

### Long term BP Goals:

» < 130/80

### 4 main classes of medications used for long term management:

» Thiazide diuretic

- Longer acting preferred

» Calcium channel blocker

- “dipines”

» ACE inhibitor

- “prils”

» Angiotensin receptor blocker (ARB)

- “sartans”

## Hypertensive Crisis

**SBP > 180 &/or DBP >120**

### Acute BP elevation associated with organ damage

- Kidney: decreased blood flow, hematuria, proteinuria
- Brain: hypertensive encephalopathy
- Heart: LVH, LVF, MI
- Eyes: retinal hemorrhages
- Vascular system: vessel damage

### Treatment:

- BP in both arms
  - R/o aortic dissection or steal syndrome
- Consider 12 Lead ECG
- ↓ BP by 25% in 1 - 2 hrs
- IV anti-hypertensives (vasodilators, diuretics, etc.)
  - Beta blockers
    - Esmolol
    - Labetalol
    - Metoprolol
  - Nitrates
    - Tridil (Nitroglycerin)
  - Calcium channel blockers
    - Nicardipine (Cardene)
    - Clevidipine (Cleviprex)
  - Hydralazine

# Aneurysms

**Definition: permanent localized dilation of aorta 1.5 times normal diameter**

- Patients will often describe “ripping” chest pain radiating to the back
- > 6 cm associated with increased risk of rupture

### Types:

- Thoracic (TAA)
- Abdominal (AAA)
- Aortic dissection
- Rupture
- Leaking

## Thoracic Aneurysm

- At risk: HTN, smoking
- Dilatation of the aorta > 50% of its normal diameter
- Goal: Prevent rupture or dissection

### Treatment:

- BP control/HR reduction
  - Beta blockers are key!
  - Reduce HR, BP & force of contraction
- Surgical repair

### BP reducing medications:

- Esmolol (Brevibloc) - short acting, beta blocker
  - Initial dose: 250 - 500 mcg/kg IV over 1 min
  - Maintenance dose: 50 – 200 mcg/kg/min IV infusion
- Labetalol (Trandate)- Blocks alpha, $B_1$ & $B_2$ receptors
  - Initial dose: 20 mg IV over 2 min
  - Follow with 20 - 80 mg IV q 10 – 15 min until BP is controlled
  - Maintenance dose: 2 mg/min IV continuous infusion; titrate up to 5 - 20 mg/min; not to exceed total dose of 300 mg
- Metoprolol
  - Dose: 5 mg IV every 2 min, up to 3 times
- Nicardipine (Cardene)
  - Calcium channel blocker
  - 5 – 15 mg/hour; minimally titrated
  - Direct arterial vasodilator
- Clevidipine (Cleviprex) can also be used

## Abdominal Aneurysm

- Pulsation in the abdomen
- Control HTN
- Surgical repair

### Signs of rupture:

- Unrelenting back pain
- Hypotension
- Tachycardia
- Shock
- Carries ~90% mortality

## Post-Op Aneurysm Repair

- BP control
- Pain management
- Closely monitor urine output
- Monitor BUN & creatinine
    - Possible ischemia d/t aortic cross-clamp
- Monitor for bleeding
- Asses extremity movement

## Aortic Dissection

- Hypertension is a risk factor
- Signs: BP difference of ≥ = 25 mm Hg between left & right arm

### Ascending aorta (Type A)

- At risk for aortic insufficiency
- Diastolic murmur
- Widened pulse pressure
- Bounding pulse
- Treatment of Type A dissection
    - Surgical repair

### Descending aorta or aortic arch (Type B)

- Often associated with atherosclerosis
- Intermittent or constant chest pain radiating to back
  - Dull pain between shoulders
- Treatment of Type B dissection
  - If dissected, administer vasodilators to keep BP controlled
  - Endovascular stenting
  - Surgical repair considered when > 6 cm in diameter

# Peripheral Arterial Disease

## Lower extremity PAD

- Greater than 60% have CAD
- Atherosclerosis
- Claudication—can be intermittent with exercise
- Limb ischemia

### Risk factors:

- Smoking
- DM
- Dyslipidemia
- HTN
- age > 70

### Monitor the 7 "P's":

- Pain
- Pallor
- Paresthesia
- Paralysis
- Pulseless
- Poor temperature
- Poor healing

### Ankle/Brachial Index (ABI)

- Arm pressure - SBP from brachial artery
- Ankle pressure - SBP from posterior tibial & dorsalis pedis arteries
- Divide ankle pressure by arm
- ABI Value > 0.9 normal
- < 0.4 severe obstruction

### Diagnostics/Treatment

- Doppler studies
- Arteriography

### Management:

**Goal is to improve perfusion!**

- Anticoagulation
  - Antiplatelet agents
  - Thrombolytic agents
- Vasodilators
- Angioplasty
- Stents
- Surgery—bypass
- Amputation

## Deep Venous Thrombosis (DVT)

- May have pain &/or swelling in affected extremity
- + Homans' sign
  - Pain in calf with abrupt dorsiflexion of the foot while the knee is flexed at 90°
  - Not a diagnostic indicator
- If shortness of breath develops, consider pulmonary embolism
- Anticoagulation usually with heparin short term, Coumadin long term
  - Direct oral anticoagulants (DOACs) are also often used
- Consider IVC filter if lower extremity DVT

You can do it!

# Cardiac Medications

| Class | Examples | Indications | Effects | Monitor for: | Watch out! |
|---|---|---|---|---|---|
| **ACE Inhibitors** | "prils" —take a "chill-pril"!<br>Class I: Captopril<br>Class II: Enalapril (Vasotec) Ramipril (Altace)<br>Benazepril (Lotensin)<br>Class III: Lisinopril | -CHF/Systolic failure<br>-AMI (EF < 40%)<br>-Anterior wall MI<br>-HTN<br>-Diabetic renal nephropathy | - Vasodilation<br>-↓ preload & afterload<br>-Prevention of myocardial remodeling<br>-Reduce progress of diabetic nephropathy | ↓ BP<br>↑ $K^+$ levels | Hypotension<br>Cough<br>Hyperkalemia<br>Angioedema<br>Renal function |
| **Beta Blockers** | "olols"<br>**Cardio-selective (blocks $B_1$):**<br>Bisoprolol, Metoprolol SR, Atenolol, Esmolol (IV), Acebutolol, Nebivolol (Bystolic)<br>**Alpha & Beta Blocking:**<br>Labetalol, Carvedilol (Coreg)<br>**Non-selective (blocks $B_1$ & $B_2$):**<br>Propranolol (Inderal), Timolol, Nadolol (Corgard), Sotalol | -HTN<br>-Secondary prevention of MI (only metoprolol tartrate or carvedilol)<br>-Cardiac arrhythmias<br>-Angina<br>-Afib<br>-CHF/Systolic failure | BB = **B**lock the heart<br>**B**reaks on the heart (↓HR)<br>-↓ HR, BP<br>-Negative inotrope, however, decreases myocardial workload<br>-↓ preload<br>-Block endogenous epi & norepi; "stress catecholamine"<br>-↓ morbidity & mortality in HF<br>-↓ arrythmias | ↓ HR<br>↓ BP<br>AV Blocks<br>Heart failure | Bradycardia<br>Hypotension<br>Signs of shock<br>Bronchospasm; Avoid in asthma!<br>Heart block<br>Avoid with cocaine use<br>**Overdose reversal:**<br>Glucagon |
| **Angiotension Receptor Blockers (ARBs)** | "sartans"<br>Valsartan, Losartan, Candesartan, Olmesartan, Telmisartan | -HTN<br>-CHF/Systolic failure<br>-Diabetic renal nephropathy<br>-Intolerance of ACE Inhibitors | -Vasodilation<br>-Decreases preload & afterload<br>-Reduces secretion of vasopressin | ↓ BP<br>↑ $K^+$ levels | Dizziness<br>Headache<br>Hyperkalemia<br>Caution: MI |

| | | | | | |
|---|---|---|---|---|---|
| **Aldosterone Blockers** | Spironolactone (Aldactone),<br>Eplerenone (Inspra) | Adjunctive therapy in heart failure | -Diuresis<br>-Blocks Na+ reabsorption<br>-↓ preload & afterload<br>-In combo with other diuretics, ↓ cardiac workload<br>-K+ sparing diuretic | $K^+$ levels | Hyperkalemia—especially when used with ACE Inhibitors or ARBs |
| **Calcium Channel Blockers (CCBs)** | "dipines" used for BP reduction!<br><br>**Dihydropyridines:** (little effect on contractility or heart rate)<br>Amlodipine, nimodipine, nicardipine (IV), Nifedipine, Felodipine<br>**Benzothiazepine class:** Diltiazem (Cardizem) - HR control<br>**Phenylalkylamine class:**<br>Verapamil (Calan) - HR control | -HTN<br>-To reduce HR<br>-SVT<br>-Afib/flutter<br>-Angina—Prinzmetal's (vasospasm)<br>-Hypertrophic CM<br>-Prevent cerebral artery vasospasm (nimodipine) | -Arterial vasodilation, ↓ afterload<br>-↓ the force of myocardial contraction<br>-Negative chronotrope<br>-Negative inotrope | ↓ HR<br>↓ BP | Heart block<br>Bradycardia<br>Reflexive tachycardia<br>Caution when used with BB<br>**Overdose:**<br>Calcium Chloride & Atropine |
| **Nitrates** | Nitroglycerin<br>Isosorbide dinitrate (Isordil),<br>Isosorbide mononitrate (Imdur) | -Angina<br>-Heart failure | -Vasodilation<br>-Venodilation | ↓ BP<br>Headaches | Hypotension |
| **Hydrazinophthalazine** | Hydralazine<br><br>*Usually prescribed in combo with isosorbide tinitrate, a BB & diuretic in heart failure | -Heart failure<br>-HTN | -Vasodilator<br>-↓ afterload | ↓ BP<br>Headaches | Reflexive tachycardia<br>MI/angina |

**Definitions:**

**Inotrope**—has an effect on contractility, positive inotrope improves contractility, negative inotrope decreases contractility.

**Chronotrope**—has an effect on heart rate, positive chronotrope increases the heart rate, negative chronotrope decreases the heart rate.

# Endocrine Review

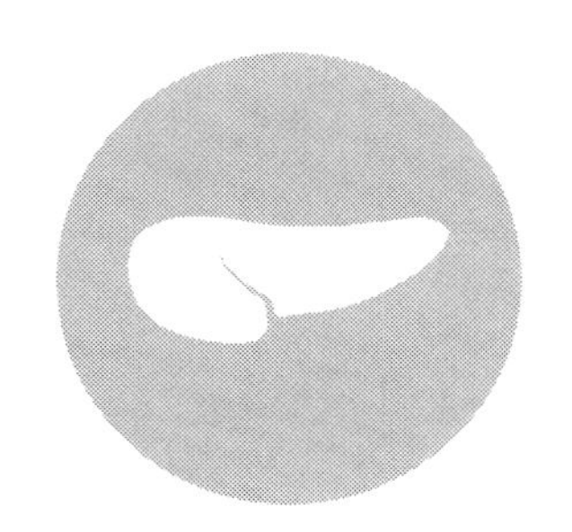

## AACN Test Plan for the Endocrine portion for the PCCN® Exam

- Diabetes mellitus
- Diabetic ketoacidosis (DKA)
- Hyperglycemia
- Hypoglycemia

# IV Fluids - Basic Concepts

## Physiologic Osmolality

- The measure of solute concentration, defined as the number of osmoles of solute per liter of solution (mOsm/L)
- Normal serum osmolality 275 – 295 mOsm/L
- **Calculation:** (FYI only)
  - $(2 \times Na^+) + (Glucose \div 18) + (BUN \div 2.8)$
  - OR, if the glucose is normal: The sodium level multiplied by 2, gives a ballpark estimate

## Osmolality of IV fluids

### Isotonic IV fluids—close to normal serum osmolality

- 0.9% Sodium Chloride (308 mOsm/L)
- Plasmalyte® (312 mOsm/L)
- Lactated Ringers (273 mOsm/L)
- When given, should stay in the vasculature

### Hypertonic Solutions (osmo higher than serum)

- D5 0.2 NS (321 mOsm/L)
- D5 ½ NS (406 mOsm/L)
- D5LR (525 mOsm/L)
- When given, will pull fluid from the cell to the vasculature
- 10% Dextrose (505 mOsm/L)
- Hypertonic Saline solutions
  - 2%, 3%, 5%, 23.4% Saline

### Hypotonic Solutions (osmo lower than serum)

- 0.45 Sodium Chloride (154 mOsm/L)
- When given, will provide cellular hydration
- $D_5W$ (252 mOsm/L)—Isotonic in the bag; the body quickly metabolizes the glucose

# Acute Hypoglycemia

- Is bad!!! Avoid it!
- Associated with higher mortality!!!
- Defined as serum glucose < 70 mg/dL
- Too much insulin in relation to glucose
- Identify cause; predisposing factors
- Frequent glucose monitoring
- Beta-blockers—Check glucose more frequently
  - Blunt the SNS
  - May not see signs of hypoglycemia

## Hypoglycemia causes:

- Too much insulin
- Vomiting
- Interrupted feedings (oral, enteral or parenteral)
- Strenuous exercise or stress (increased metabolic needs)
- Excessive ETOH
- Adrenal insufficiency
- Severe liver disease
- Pregnancy

## Hypoglycemia Symptoms: Cardiovascular

**Initial symptoms observed due to activation of the sympathetic nervous system**

- Palpitations
- Tachycardia
- Diaphoresis
- Pallor
- Cool skin
- Piloerection ("goose bumps")
- Irritability

### Hypoglycemia Symptoms: Neurologic

- Blurred vision
- Slurred speech
- Weakness
- Headache
- Difficulty concentrating
- Confusion
- Fatigue
- Diplopia
- Anxiety
- Tremors
- Staggering gate

**Concerns when blood glucose is < 50 mg/dL:**

- Seizures

**Concerns when blood glucose is < 20 mg/dL:**

- Coma

### Hypoglycemia Treatment

- If conscious:
  - 4 oz. juice
  - 10 – 15 grams of Carbohydrates
  - Glucose tablets or gel
- If unconscious with IV access:
  - 0.5 to 1 amp of Dextrose 50%
  - Consider 5 - 10% Dextrose in water infusion
- If unconscious without IV access:
  - Glucagon 0.5 – 1 mg IM
- Provide longer acting carbohydrate once stabilized

# Metabolic Syndrome

- Estimated 25% of the US population
  - 40% incidence age > 60
- High risk for developing CV disease & stroke

**Any 2 of the following:**

» Dyslipidemia

- Elevated triglycerides > 150 mg/dL
- Low HDL < 40 in males, < 50 in female

» Hypertension

- Elevated BP: SBP > 130 or DBP > 85

» Hyperglycemia

- Fasting blood glucose > 100 or diagnosed Type 2 DM

» Abdominal obesity

- Waistline > 40 inches men, > 35 inches women

# Hyperglycemia & Diabetes Mellitus

» Fasting BG > 126 mg/dL & $A_1C \geq 6.5\%$

» Defect in insulin secretion, insulin resistance or both

**4 Categories of Diabetes Mellitus:**

» **Type 1:** Beta cell destruction resulting in **absolute** insulin **deficiency**

» **Type 2:** Insulin secretory defect; insulin **resistance** resulting in **relative** insulin deficiency

» **"Other":** due to other causes; genetic, medication induced

» **Gestational Diabetes:** due to pregnancy

**The pancreas is an endocrine gland:**

» **Alpha cells** produce glucagon

» **Beta cells** produce insulin

» **Delta cells** produce somatostatin

## $HgbA_1C$

» Estimates the effectiveness of diabetes mellitus therapy

» Glucose & hemoglobin have a high affinity for each other

» Reflective of glucose levels over 3 month period of time

» Normal value 4 - 5.6% (non-diabetic)

- » 6 - 7%: average glucose range 100 - 150 mg/dL
- » > 7%: indicative of poorly controlled glucose levels
  - Doesn't necessarily mean the patient is non-compliant
  - In patients with multiple co-morbid conditions, the goal $A_1C$ may be higher

### Limitations of $HgbA_1C$:

- » African Americans have greater glycation than other ethnicities
- » Anemia

# Insulin

### Action of Insulin

- » Drives glucose, water & potassium into cells
- » Regular insulin (IV) onset of action: about 5 – 10 min
- » Regular insulin (SQ) onset of action: 30 min
  - Peak: 1 – 3 hours
  - Effects last up to 12 hours

**Insulin at a glance:**

| Type | Brand Name | Onset | Peak | Duration |
|---|---|---|---|---|
| Rapid-acting | Humalog<br>Novolog<br>Apidra | 5 - 15 minutes | 1 - 3 hours | 3 - 5 hours |
| Short-acting | Regular (R) | 30 minutes - 1 hour | 1 - 3 hours | Up to 12 hours |
| Intermediate-acting | NPH (N) | 1.5 - 4 hours | 4 - 12 hours | Up to 24 hours |
| Long-acting | Lantus<br>Levemir | 0.8 - 4 hours | Minimal peak | Up to 24 hours |

# Diabetic Ketoacidosis (DKA) & Hyperosmolar Hyperglycemic Syndrome (HHS)

## Always look for a cause in DKA & HHS:

- Type 1 DM (DKA)
- Undiagnosed Type 1 DM (20% of DKA cases)
- Stress
- Illness/Infection
- Trauma
- Surgery
- Non-compliance
- Pancreatitis
- Pregnancy
- Cushing's Syndrome
- Hyperthyroidism
- Diet
- Medications
  - Thiazide diuretics
  - Glucocorticoids (e.g. prednisone)
  - Diazoxide (hyperstat)
  - Phenytoin
  - Sympathomimetics (e.g. epinephrine, norepinephrine)

## Diabetic Ketoacidosis (DKA):

- Lack of insulin leaves too much circulating glucose
  - Drives up the serum osmolality
- Osmotic diuresis leads to profound water loss (polyuria)
- Leads to glucosuria, dehydration & electrolyte imbalance

## Metabolism issues associated with insulin deficiency:

- Accelerated gluconeogenesis
- Glycogenolysis
- Decreased glucose utilization
- Increased lipolysis
- Decreased lipogenesis
- Abundant free fatty acids are converted to **ketone bodies**

## Nursing assessment in DKA

- The "3 P's":
  - Polyuria (early), oliguria –(late)
  - Polydipsia (due to profound water loss)
  - Polyphagia (due to ketosis/fat burning)
- Neurologic:
  - Headache
  - Decreased deep tendon reflexes (DTRs); sluggish & limp
  - Visual disturbances
  - Hypo/hyperthermia
  - Decreased level of consciousness (LOC); may advance to coma
- Cardiovascular:
  - Tachycardia
  - Decreased preload (due to dehydration)
  - Hypotension (severe cases)
- Pulmonary:
  - Kussmaul's breathing, rapid shallow breathing (blowing off ketones)
  - Acetone/fruity odor to breath
- GI:
  - Nausea, vomiting
  - Abdominal pain
  - Weight loss

## Laboratory findings in DKA

- Hyperglycemic crisis (BG 300 - 800 mg/dL)
- Metabolic acidosis
  - Low pH: if > 7.0 let the patient self-correct, if < 6.9 – consider sodium bicarbonate
  - Serum bicarbonate level is often < 20 mEq/L
  - Anion gap > 15; often in the 20s
- Elevated serum & urine ketones
- Electrolyte imbalances:
  - Increased $K^+$ (acidosis causes $K^+$ to shift out of cell)
  - Decreased $Na^+$ & $Ca^{++}$

## Anion gap: Normal < 11 - 12

- Difference between primary measured cations ($Na^+$ & $K^+$) and the primary measured anions ($Cl^-$ & $HCO_3^-$) in serum
- If the gap is >12; often associated with metabolic acidosis

### Here's an easy acronym to remember causes of **metabolic acidosis**:

**M**: Methanol

**U**: Uremia

**D**: DKA

**P**: Propylene glycol

**I**: Isoniazid

**L**: Lactic acidosis

**E**: Ethylene glycol

**S**: Salicylates

## Management of Diabetic Ketoacidosis (DKA)

- A fluid deficit should be calculated
  - It's often ~ 50 – 100 mL/kg
- Depending on the calculated fluid deficit:
  - Administer 1 - 3 liters of IV fluid during the first hour
  - Administer 1 L during the second hour
  - Administer 1 L during the following 2 hours
  - Administer 1 L every 4 hours, depending on the degree of dehydration
- Fluid Management—DKA
  - 0.9% Saline or Lactated Ringers (isotonic)
  - Add dextrose to the IV fluids when BG reaches 250 mg/dL (i.e. D5.45)**
  - Then, 0.45% saline @ 250 - 500 mL/hour (hypotonic) for cellular hydration
  - Quick tip: Often this last step is skipped if the patient is able to drink water
  - Water is hypotonic and will provide cellular hydration

## Insulin Management—DKA

- **Insulin (Regular)**
  - Begin infusion at 0.1 units/kg/hour
  - FYI: Often hospitals use an algorithm-based approach to manage insulin
  - Insulin infusion goal: ↓ glucose SLOWLY!!!

- Do not drop BG by more than 50 - 100 mg/dL per hour
  - Please note: dropping by 100 mg/dL is on the rapid side!
  - Most protocols shoot closer to 50 mg/dL
- Assess blood glucose every 1 - 2 hours until goal is reached

» Transition to subcutaneous insulin when:

1) The anion gap is corrected
2) Ketone body production has ceased (assess serum ketones)
3) The glucose is generally less than 200 mg/dL

- Continue to run the insulin infusion for 1 – 2 hours after resuming subcutaneous insulin
  - Prevents patient from going back into DKA

## Electrolyte management—DKA

» **Potassium**

- Serum $K^+$ is initially elevated in about 22% of cases, normal in about 74% of cases
- But, there is a total body potassium depletion
- Average deficit is 3 – 5 mEq/L
- Transcellular $K^+$ shifts with insulin

» **Sodium**

- Dehydration is not reflected in $Na^+$ levels
- Glucose has a dilutional effect on $Na^+$
- For every 100 mg/dL ↑ in glucose, the $Na^+$ decreases by 1.6 – 2.0 mEq/L

» **Phosphate**

- Depletion is common
- Do not replace unless $PO_4$ < 1.0 mg/dL
- Replacement has little impact on outcome in DKA

» **Magnesium**

- Often depleted

## Acidosis—DKA

» $K^+$ & pH have an inverse relationship

» For every 0.1 ↓ in pH, the serum potassium can ↑ by 0.6 mEq/L

**Quick tip:** It's concerning when a patient presents with normal or low potassium levels in the setting of DKA. When insulin & fluids are given there is lots of intracellular shifting and the patient may become severely hypokalemic!

Also, ALWAYS know what the patient's potassium level is prior to administering insulin!

## Hyperosmolar Hyperglycemic Syndrome (HHS)

- aka "HHNS", "HHNK", "non-ketotic hyperosmolar hyperglycemia"
- Type 2 DM
  - Precipitated by physiologic stress (i.e. trauma, infection, etc.)
  - Non-compliance
  - Look for a cause!!!
  - Review many of the same reasons a patient develops DKA!

### Clinical signs of HHS:

- **Absence of ketones**
  - Have enough endogenous insulin to prevent ketosis
- Glucose is often > 600, can be >1000 mg/dL
- Polyuria—early sign, then oliguria
  - Urine gets concentrated
  - Persistent loss of glucose in the urine
  - Osmotic diuresis
    - Serum osmo > 330 mOs/L due to dehydration
  - Profound **hypovolemia**
- Altered mental status
- Takes days to weeks to develop

## HHS—Treatment:

- Volume replacement
  - A fluid deficit should be calculated to gauge fluid replacement needs
  - Start with isotonic solution (0.9 Saline or LR)
  - May need colloids if in hypovolemic shock
  - Add dextrose to IV fluids when glucose is lowered to 250 - 300 mg/dL
  - Last step: Hypotonic fluids for cellular hydration
    - 0.45% Saline or $D_5W$ (when euvolemic & osmo < 320 mOs/L)
- Insulin (Regular)
  - Normalize glucose gradually—will not require as much insulin as DKA
  - Monitor serum glucose hourly
  - +/- Bolus followed by infusion (mixed opinions about bolus)

| Recap of DKA vs. HHS: | | |
|---|---|---|
| | DKA | HHNS |
| Glucose level | 300 – 800 | 600 - 2000 |
| Ketones present? | Yes | No |
| Acid/base | Metabolic acidosis | Normal/mild acidosis |
| Anion gap present? | Yes (> 15) | No |
| Osmolality | 295 – 330 | 330 – 450 |
| Fluid deficit | > 5 L | > 10 L |
| Type of Diabetic | Type 1 | Type 2 |
| Mortality | 1% | 5 – 10% |

# Syndrome of Inappropriate Antidiuretic Hormone (SIADH) and Diabetes Insipidus (DI)

## Anti-Diuretic Hormone (ADH)

- » Purpose of ADH: Maintain fluid balance
- » ADH formed in the hypothalamus (brain)
- » Released from the posterior pituitary
- » Has vasopressor qualities

## Syndrome of Inappropriate Anti-Diuretic Hormone (SIADH)

- » **Acronym: S**wimming **I**n **ADH**; too much **ADH**
- » Water intoxication (kidneys hold onto water & often dilute $Na^+$)

### Signs:

- » **Severe Dilutional Hyponatremia**
  - Serum $Na^+ < 120$ mEq/L
- » Decreased serum osmolality (< 280 mOsm/L) – d/t dilution
- » Urine osmolality > 100 mOsm/L (urine is concentrated)
- » Decreased urine output

### Causes of SIADH:

- » Infection
- » Any pulmonary cause – pneumonia, COPD, PE
- » CNS insults – CVA, ICH, head trauma
- » Variety of carcinomas/tumors
- » Recent surgery (stress)

### Complications of SIADH:

- » Severe dilutional hyponatremia
- » Seizure activity
- » Cerebral edema

### Treatment of SIADH:

- » Safety!!!
- » Remedy the problem
- » Fluid/free water restriction
- » Hypertonic saline (i.e. 2%, 3%)
- » Assess for fluid overload
  - Diuretics (loop diuretics like furosemide)
- » Sodium correction:
  - Needs to be slow!
  - Do not exceed 0.5 mEq/L per hour or 12 mEq/L per day
  - If corrected too quickly, can cause demyelination syndrome (permanent nerve damage)
  - Do not exceed plasma $Na^+$ > 130 mEq/L with replacement

## Diabetes Insipidus (DI)

- » Sip & pis (Sorry, but it's an easy way to remember!)
- » Lack of ADH
- » Failure of ADH release from the posterior pituitary
- » Water loss up to 20 L/day
- » Can be neurogenic or nephrogenic in nature

### Common causes (neurogenic most common):

- » TBI
- » Hypoxic-Ischemic encephalopathy
- » Meningitis
- » Brain death
- » Dilantin
- » Tumors
- » Can also see nephrogenic causes

## DI Symptoms:

- Polyuria
  - Dilute urine (water loss)
  - Urine specific gravity < 1.005 (dilute)
  - Urine osmolality < 200 mOsm/L (dilute)
- Extreme polydipsia
- Elevated BUN (d/t dehydration)
- Low serum ADH levels
- Serum osmolality elevated (> 295 mOsm/L)
- Serum $Na^+$ > 145 mEq/L (d/t $H_2O$ loss)
- Low urine osmolality (50 – 200)
- Low urine specific gravity (< 1.005)

## DI Treatment:

- Replace ADH: (IV, IM, PO, SQ, intranasal)
- Desmopressin (DDAVP)
  - IV/SQ: 2 – 4 mcg/day SQ
  - PO: 0.05 mg q 12 hours
  - Intranasal: 10 – 40 mcg/day
- Fluid replacement
- Calculate & replace the free water deficit
- Correct fluid deficit slowly over 2 – 3 days
  - Limits risk of cerebral edema

You can do it!

# Gastrointestinal Review

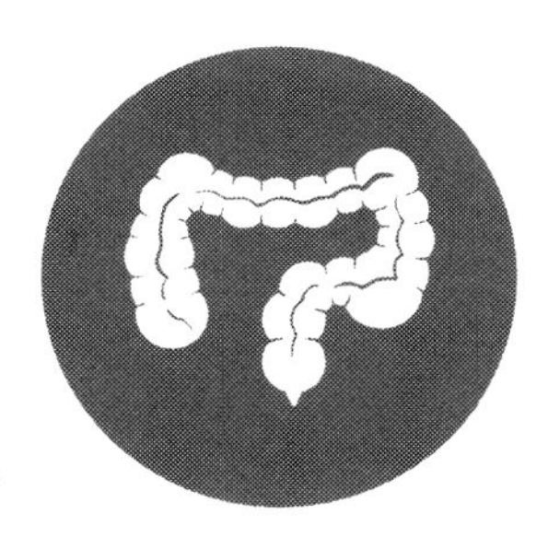

## AACN Test Plan for the Gastrointestinal portion of the PCCN® Exam

- Functional GI disorders (i.e. obstruction, ileus, diabetic gastroparesis, gastroesophageal reflux, irritable bowel syndrome)
- GI bleed (lower & upper)
- GI infections (C. difficile)
- GI surgeries (resections, Esophagogastrectomy, bariatric)
- Hepatic disorders (cirrhosis, hepatitis, portal hypertension)
- Ischemic bowel
- Malnutrition (failure to thrive, malabsorption disorders)
- Pancreatitis

# Abdominal assessment

**Proper order:**

- » Inspection
- » Auscultation
- » Percussion
- » Palpation—always last!
- » "Look, listen, feel"

## Small Intestine

- » Pyloric sphincter to the cecum
- » 18 to 20 feet in length
- » Lumen have villi, fingerlike projections to ↑ surface area
  - Aids in digestion

**3 segments:**

- » Duodenum - 10 inches in length
- » Jejunum - 8 feet in length
- » Ileum - 12 feet
- » Major role is digestion & absorption
  - Carbohydrates
  - Fats
  - Protein/Amino acids
  - Water
  - Electrolytes

## Large Intestine

- » 5 to 6 feet in length, 2.5 in diameter
- » Extends from the ileum to the anus
- » Lumen do not have villi like the small intestines
- » Responsible for absorption of $H_2O$, electrolytes & elimination of wastes

### Three sections:

- Cecum
- Rectum
- Colon
  - Subdivided: Ascending, transverse, descending, sigmoid

### Large Intestine Function

- Absorbs 800 – 900 ml fluid
- Bacteria cause formation of gas
- Synthesize vitamin K, thiamine, riboflavin, B12, folic acid, biotin & nicotinic acid
- Main aerobic bacteria is E. coli

# Intestinal Infarction

- 20% of the cardiac output goes to the intestines after eating
- Infarction is rare d/t collateral blood flow

### Two main types of infarction:

- Occlusive:
  - Embolus or thrombosis to the superior mesenteric artery or major vessel
  - Adequate C.O.
- Non-occlusive:
  - Associated with decreased C.O. or BP
  - At risk: patients with atherosclerosis, heart failure, low C.O. or any shock state
  - Ischemia is secondary to overall low perfusion

### Symptoms of intestinal infarction:

- Abdominal pain***
- Vomiting
- Abdominal distention
- Diarrhea
- Fever
- Physiologic changes:
  - Ischemia
  - Bowel edema
  - Necrosis
  - Can lead to perforation or peritonitis

### Intestinal Infarction Diagnosis:

- History & clinical presentation
- Rule out other causes
- CT scan—assess for free air (perforation)
- Radiographic angiography
  - Assess for embolus or thrombus
- Surgery
  - Assess for ischemic or infarcted bowel (more difficult)
  - May need resection with colostomy or ileostomy

### Labs:

- Nonspecific
- Leukocytosis
- Elevated LDH, amylase
- Follow serial lactate levels
  - Elevation is a sign of tissue hypoxia
- May see metabolic acidosis in shock states

### Treatment:

- Adequate resuscitation
- Both:
  - Manage pain
  - Decompress the stomach, gastric tube
  - Resect infarcted bowl

- Occlusive:
  - Angiogram—clot lysis
  - Anticoagulation
  - Thrombolytic therapy if present within 8 hours of onset of symptoms
- Non-occlusive:
  - Vasodilator therapy to dilate the mesenteric arterial bed
  - Surgery—resect infarcted bowel
  - ↑ C.O. and perfusion to gut
    - +Inotrope

# Bowel obstruction

## Causes:

- Adhesions from previous surgery
- Incarcerated hernia
- Tumors
  - Can cause partial or complete obstruction
- Ulcers
- Ileus
- Opiates
- Infections
  - Abscesses
  - Diverticulitis
- Volvulus
  - Small intestines
- Intussusception

## Signs & symptoms

- Duodenal or proximal small bowel:
  - Depends on location & etiology
  - **Vomiting
  - Crampy, epigastric pain
  - Dehydrated
  - High pitched bowl sounds
  - Hypokalemia
- Distal small bowel or large bowel:
  - Vague abdominal pain
  - Decreased passing of stool or gas
  - Constipation
  - Vomiting (late—hours to days after, vomit fecal matter)

### Both:

- Decreased PO intake
- Fluid trapped in intestinal loops
- **Early**—bowel sounds are increased, **late**—decreased

### Diagnosis:

- Clinical presentation & history
- Abdominal radiograph
  - Dilated loops of bowel
- Endoscopy
- CT scan
- Upper GI
- Abdominal ultrasound

### Treatment:

- Adequate fluids
- Electrolyte replacement
- Monitor for ileus
  - NG tube! (removes air & decompresses stomach)
- Surgery if suspected:
  - Adhesions
  - Incarcerated hernia
  - Diverticuli
  - Volvulus
- Antibiotics (if indicated)

## Gastric perforation

- Rare, can be fatal
- Stomach, duodenum, appendix, colon
- Ulcerative Colitis
- Penetrating trauma/wounds
- "Rigid" abdomen (guarding)
- Leakage of intestinal content into the peritoneum
- Systemic inflammatory response (SIRS) & infection
  - Tachycardia, tachypnea
  - Fever, leukocytosis & severe abdominal pain
- Elevated Hgb/Hct
  - Hemo-concentrated d/t dehydration

### Diagnosis:

- Clinical presentation
- Abdominal films
    - Free air in abdomen
- Exploratory lap—need to go to the OR!

### Treatment:

- Surgery
    - Abdominal washout
- Adequate volume resuscitation
- Antibiotics
- Gastric decompression
- Nutritional support

# Acute GI Hemorrhage

### Upper GI Bleeding:

- Make up 80% of GIB
- Higher mortality
- Stomach or small intestine
- Ulcers/erosion
- NSAIDs
- Excess acid production
- Stress
- Esophagogastric varicies
- Chronic portal hypertension
- AV Malformations within the intestines
- Mallory-Weiss tear
- Tumor/cancer

### Symptoms:

- Abdominal pain—upper quadrants
- Pain worse after eating
- Offenders: ETOH, aspirin, spicy food
- Vomit blood—bright red or coffee ground
- Blood in stool (dark)
    - Dumping syndrome—may have bright red stool
- Can go into shock

## Diagnosis:

- ***Endoscopy
- Active hemorrhage may require angiography (embolization)

## Treatment:

- Maintain optimal hemodynamics
- Transfusions (if Hgb < 7 - 8 mg/dL)
- Clotting factors
  - FFP
  - Platelets
  - Cryoprecipitate
- $H_2$ blockers or PPIs (IV, then PO)
  - Reduces the risk of mucosal lining damage
- Vasopressin infusion
  - 0.1 – 0.8 units/min
  - Constricts the splanchnic vascular bed
  - Use cautiously in CAD
  - Decreases portal htn
- Octreotide acetate (Sandostatin)
  - 50 - 150 mcg SQ BID/TID
  - Infusion: 25 - 50 mcg/hr x 24 - 48 hrs

## Lower GI Bleeding:

- Distal small intestine & colon
- 5 Types:
  - Anatomic
    - Diverticuli—outpouchings in intestine
    - Lack of fiber in diet
    - Can become infected & bleed
  - Vascular
    - Arteriovenous malformations (AVMs)
  - Inflammatory
  - Neoplastic
    - Colon tumors
    - Polyps
  - Infectious
    - C.Diff

**Diagnosis & Treatment:**

- Colonoscopy
- Barium enema
- Endoscopic or surgical removal
- Severe cases may require embolization or surgery (resection)
- Endoscopic laser, thermal or electrical coagulation

# Gastrointestinal Trauma

**Blunt "closed" Trauma:**

- Motor vehicle collision ("seat belt sign")
- Sports injury
- Risk of bleeding or contusion

**Organs at risk:**

- Spleen
- Kidney
- Pancreas
- Duodenum
- Liver

**Penetrating Trauma:**

- Stab wounds, gunshot wounds (GSW)
- High risk of bleeding
- Risk of peritonitis

**Organs at risk:**

- Liver
- Stomach
- Colon
- Spleen

### FAST Exam

- **F**ocused **A**ssessment with **S**onography for **T**rauma
- Ultrasound screen for blood around heart & abdominal cavity

### Diagnosis:

- CT scan** (gold standard for trauma)
- Identify other organs injured
- Can detect hemorrhage, hematomas, ruptures, lacerations

### Treatment:

- Surgery if penetrating trauma or active bleeding
- Liver or splenic injury may require arterial embolization
- Tranexamic Acid (TXA)
  - 1 Gram given pre-hospital to promote fibrinolysis (clotting)
- 1:1:1 blood replacement if active bleeding
  - PRBCs, FFP, Platelets
  - Cryoprecipitate if fibrinogen < 100 mg/L
  - Caution with crystalloids – give sparingly
  - Closely monitor Hgb & coags
- Antibiotics for penetrating trauma

# Intra-Abdominal Hypertension (IAH)

- Increased intra-abdominal pressure from 3rd spacing of fluids
- Associated with fluid resuscitation
- Inflammation
- Capillary leak

## Who's at risk?

- Up to 30% of trauma patients
- Over 35% of major abdominal surgery
- Up to 8% of critically ill patients

## Signs/Symptoms of abdominal hypertension:

- Abdominal distention
- Decreased urine output
- Intra-abdominal pressure (IAP) > 25 mm Hg
  - Normal bladder pressure is 5 – 10 mm Hg
- Abdominal perfusion pressure:
  - MAP minus bladder pressure (IAP)
  - > 60 mm Hg (ideal)
- Respiratory compromise:
  - Shortness of breath, increased respiratory rate
  - Pressure on the diaphragm
  - Difficult ventilation
- Hemodynamic effects:
  - Decreased venous return due to pressure on IVC
  - Decreased C.O./BP
  - Increased afterload
  - Increased preload

## Monitoring/ Treatment:

- Assess bladder pressure via bladder catheter
- If IAP > 25 mm Hg – indication of Intra-Abdominal Compartment Syndrome (IACS)
  - Must go to the ICU!
- Decompressive laparotomy; abdomen is left open (extreme cases)— usually in the ICU
- Monitor for organ ischemia
- Follow lactate levels

# Hepatic failure

- Acute, Chronic or Acute on Chronic
- 75 - 90% of hepatocytes lost before failure occurs

## Functions of the liver:

- Filters toxins
- Filters $NH_3$ – ammonia
- Synthesize plasma proteins
- Albumin & coagulation factors

## Causes of failure:

- Hepatitis
- Fatty liver
- ETOH
- Starvation
- Obesity
- Diabetes
- Advanced cirrhosis
- Hepatic tumors
- Fulminant
- Viral
- Toxin induced (acetaminophen, ecstasy)
- Ischemia (shock, MODS)

# Acute Hepatic Injury

## Etiology:

- Inflammation
- Hepatic necrosis
- No prior liver failure
- Encephalopathy & jaundice
- No portal hypertension

## Causes:

- 15 – 20% are from herbal & dietary supplements
- Anabolic steroids
- Green tea extract
- Drug induced (DILI)***
  - Acetaminophen most common
- Fulminant
  - Viral
  - Acute hepatitis
  - Autoimmune hepatitis
  - Cholangitis
  - Toxin induced (ecstasy)

## Clinical features:

- Jaundice PLUS
  - Bilirubin > 2x's the upper limit of normal
- ↑ aminotransferase
  - 3 x's the upper limit of normal = bad prognosis
- Mortality 10 – 50% without transplant
- Acetaminophen is the #1 cause of DILI
- Only ½ ODs are intentional
  - Chronic supratherapeutic acetaminophen use
  - Chronic acetaminophen use can be more toxic vs. acute ingestion
  - Patients with liver disease should limit acetaminophen to ≤ 2 grams/day
  - Surprisingly, concomitant ETOH use doesn't ↑ hepatic toxicity risk:
    - It may be somewhat protective because both compete for enzyme
    - Decreases toxic metabolite
- N-Acetylcysteine (NAC, Mucomyst) is the antidote

# Chronic Hepatic Failure/Advanced Cirrhosis

## Etiology/Symptoms:

- Scarring, fibrosis
- Hepatic parenchymal cells destroyed, replaced with fibrotic tissue
- Constriction of blood flow leads to portal hypertension
- Encephalopathy
- Hepato-renal syndrome
- High risk of developing liver carcinoma

## Causes:

- Chronic ETOH***
- Fatty Liver
  - Starvation, obesity, diabetes
- Advanced Cirrhosis
- Hepatitis
- Hepatic tumors

## Physical symptoms:

- Atrophied muscles
- Splenomegaly
- Distended abdomen (ascites)
- Tissue paper thin skin
- Hemorrhoids
- Jaundice
- Lower extremity edema
- Spider angiomas

## Labs: (know these!)

- ↓ Albumin, protein
- ↓ Platelet count, fibrinogen
- ↓ $Na^+$, $K^+$, $Mg^{++}$, $Ca^{++}$, glucose
- ↑ RBCs, ↑/ ↓ WBCs
- ↑ Hepatic Transaminases
- ↑ AST, ALT, LDH, alkaline phosphatase

- ↑ AST/ALT ratio > 1 = chronic failure
- ↑ PTT/PT/INR
- ↑ Lactate
- ↑ Bilirubin
- ↑ Ammonia
- ↑ Aldosterone & ADH
  - Contribute to fluid retention

## Clinical Presentation:

- Hypotension
- GI Bleed
- Weight loss
- Poor appetite
- Ascites
  - Hydrostatic pressure pushes fluid into abdominal space
- Shortness of breath
  - Pressure from ascites push on diaphragm
- Chronic low albumin level
- Portal HTN
- Poor renal perfusion
- Jaundice (↑ bilirubin)
  - Usually scleral first

**Neuro:**

- Lethargic
- Slow to respond
- Slurred speech
- Decreased LOC
- Asterixis
  - Flapping hands
- Hepatic encephalopathy
- Cerebral edema
- Increased ICPs
- Seizures
- Coma

## Cirrhosis Diagnosis:

- Ultrasound
  - Assess for portal hypertension & nodules
- Liver biopsy

## Treatment:

- Treat the cause
- Eliminate cause (ETOH)
- Symptom management
- Evaluate for liver transplant

## Ascites Management:

- Low $Na^+$ diet
- Little evidence to protein restrict unless encephalopathic
  - Many patients are malnourished
- Fluid restriction
  - 1.5 L/day
- Diuretics
  - Aldosterone antagonists (spironolactone)
  - Loop diuretics
- Paracentesis
  - Not first line treatment
  - Issues with re-accumulation

## Nursing Care:

- Measure abdominal girth
- Daily weights
- Monitor labs
- Monitor for hepato-renal syndrome (HRS)
  - Oliguria
  - Decreased urine $Na^+$
  - Increased BUN/Creatinine
- Monitor for bleeding
  - Vitamin K abnormalities
- Monitor for sepsis
  - Spontaneous Baterial Peritonitis (SBP)
  - Translocation of bacteria from GI tract to blood stream
  - Lactulose may be protective against SBP
- Monitor neuro changes & LOC
- Drug clearance
  - Caution with sedatives (especially benzodiazepines)

- » If ammonia elevated—administer lactulose
  - Poorly absorbed sugar
  - Decreases bowel pH
  - Ammonia excreted in stool
- » Nutrition
  - Enteral or parenteral nutrition if unable to take PO
- » Monitor respiratory status
  - Pressure on diaphragm from ascites
  - Paracenteris if SOB not resolving with diuretics

# Esophageal Varices

## Clinical Presentation:

- » Dilated, engorged sub-mucosal veins in the mid to distal esophagus
- » Caused by chronic portal hypertension
- » 30% mortality associated with a bleed
- » Elevated liver enzymes, bilirubin, coag times (PT/INR)
- » Quickly go into hypovolemic, hemorrhagic shock

## Treatment:

- » Control bleeding
- » Correct coags
- » Airway protection
- » Hemodynamic support
- » Endoscopic banded ligation
- » Sclerotherapy
  - High incidence of re-bleed
- » Achieve hemostasis:
  - Octreotide (Sandostatin)
    - ▹ Long acting – continue for up to 5 days post bleed
    - ▹ Reduces portal venous pressure
    - ▹ Reduces risk of re-bleeding
    - ▹ Similar to the hormone Somatostatin
    - ▹ Inhibits the release of glucagon, which is a splanchnic vasodilator

» Vasopressin infusion
  * 0.2 – 0.8 units/min
  * Reduces portal pressure

» Beta blockers (propranolol)

» Nitrates

» For bleeding, esophageal balloon (done in ICU)
  * Tamponade bleeding varices

» Transjugular Intrahepatic Portosystemic Shunting (TIPS)
  * Done in Interventional Radiology
  * Blood directed from the portal vein to the hepatic vein to relieve pressure in the portal system
  * Encephalopathy may develop or worsen
  * Higher risk uncontrolled bleeding

# Pancreatitis

» Pancreas is composed of head, body & tail

» Endocrine gland
  * Secretion of insulin
  * Secretion of glucagon

» Exocrine gland
  * Release digestive enzymes
  * 10% of pancreatic enzymes must be present to prevent malabsorption

## Pancreatic enzymes

» Pancreatic amylase
  * Alpha amylase released in saliva
  * Breaks down carbohydrates
  * Breaks down raw & cooked starches

» Lipase
  * Digest fats
  * Bile salts are essential for this!!!

## Acute Pancreatitis

» Acute, local inflammation; triggers systemic inflammation

» Enzymatic auto-digestion of the pancreas

» Triggers systemic inflammation
  * SIRS
  * Capillary leak
  * Vasodilation

- Digestive enzymes are activated prior to release from the pancreas
- Obstruction of the pancreatic duct can lead to activation of digestive enzymes
- 2 most common causes of duct obstruction:
  - ETOH
    - Chronic ETOH leads to structural changes to the pancreas
  - Gall stones

## Clinical Presentation:

- Pain—upper abdomen, often radiates to the back
- Tender, distended abdomen
- Bowel sounds decreased or absent
- Nausea, vomiting
- Fever
- Tachycardia
- Hypotension
- Pulmonary issues
  - Pleural effusions
    - Left-sided or bilateral due to inflamed pancreas near left diaphragm
    - Elevated hemi-diaphragm
  - Atelectasis
- Pulmonary infiltrates
  - Monitor for increasing $O_2$ needs
  - Monitor for ARDS!!!

## Necrotizing Pancreatitis—most severe form

- Necrosis of pancreas, peri-pancreatic tissue & fat
- Hemorrhage
- S/S Hypovolemic shock
- Sequestration of fluids in the peritoneum
- Cullen's sign—ecchymosis around umbilicus
- Grey-Turner's—flank ecchymosis
- May appear within 1 - 2 weeks with hemorrhagic pancreatitis

## Diagnosis of Acute Pancreatitis:

» Labs

» CT scan

- Caution with IV contrast; high risk for kidney injury

» Ultrasound

- Assess for gall stones & pancreatic fluid collections
- If gallstone obstruction—ERCP (endoscopic retrograde cholangiopancreatography)

» MRI

- Visual fluid collections or masses

## Lab findings:

» Elevation of amylase***

- Elevates within 24 hours
- Many times over 500
- Can return to normal within 3 to 5 days after onset
- Not a marker of severity
- Elevated urinary amylase

» Elevated lipase

- Stays elevated longer than amylase

» Hypocalcemia

- Follow ionized calcium
- Calcium binds with fatty acids from necrotic fat
- Low albumin

» Hypokalemia & hypomagnesemia

» H/H—may be increased or decreased (especially later)

» Leukocytosis

» Hypoxemia

» Hypoalbuminemia

» Hyperglycemia

- Will likely need insulin

» Steatorrhea

## Easy acronym to remember highlights of pancreatitis:

**P** = $PaO_2$ (< 60, ARDS)

**A** = Age (> 55 y.o.)

**N** = Neutrophils (Increased WBCs)

**C** = Calcium (Hypocalcemia)

**R** = Renal function (Increased BUN)

**E** = Enzymes (Elevated ALT/LDH)

**A** = Albumin (hypoalbuminemia)

**S** = Sugar (Hyperglycemia)

## Treatment

» Supportive
- Multi-system organ failure
- Pain management

» Rest the pancreas

» Nutritional support, feed as soon as possible
- Feeding tube often placed past the duodenum/ pancreatic duct
- NG tube if ileus is present
- Parenteral nutrition if necessary

## Nursing interventions, monitor for:

» Respiratory compromise
- Pulmonary effusions
- Atelectasis
- ARDs

» Hypovolemia
- Ensure adequate volume resuscitation
- Careful not to fluid overload

# General nutrition in critically ill patients

## American Society for Parenteral & Enteral Nutrition (ASPEN) Guidelines

### If not taking PO nutrition:

- » Caloric goals ~ 20 – 25 kcal/kg
  - Try to achieve the kcal goal by day 4 – 8
- » Optimize protein 1.2 – 2 grams/kg/day
- » Enteral nutrition preferred over parenteral
  - Can supplement with parenteral if not meeting goals
- » Start feedings early at a lower rate
- » Monitor for refeeding syndrome
  - Can develop within 4 days after prolonged NPO with introduction of nutrition
  - Watch phosphate levels – may drop!
  - Monitor for other electrolyte imbalances & muscle weakness
- » Keep glucose < 180 mg/dL

# Clostridium difficile

- » Most common and most costly healthcare associated infection—HIGH recurrence rate!!
- » Gram (+) spore forming anaerobe
- » How patients get it:
  - C.diff is normal flora! However, antibiotic usage alters the balance of gut flora →
  - C.diff toxin enters & destroys integrity of the epithelial layer of intestinal lining →
  - Bacterial translocation leads to infection

### Treatment options:

- Vancomycin
  - PO/PFT ONLY (IV treats completely different infections)
  - 125 - 500 mg q 6 hours x 10 days
  - Never IV!!!
- Fidaxomicin (Dificid)
  - 200 mg BID x 10 days
  - ↓ in recurrence compared to Vancomycin
  - Common to extend treatment 5 - 7 days after broad spectrum antibiotic course ends

### For recurrent C. Diff infections:

- Strongest recommendation—Fecal Microbiota Transplant (FMT)
  - Capsules (nicknamed "crapsules" by many people... honestly though, I'd take them if I had C. diff!)
  - NG tube
  - Colonoscopy
  - Over 90% effective for cure
- Fidaxomicin x 10 days
- Vancomycin x 10 days, if treated with metronidazole initially

# Bariatric Surgery

### Types of Procedures:

- Adjustable Gastric Banding
- Gastric Sleeve (aka Vertical Sleeve Gastrectomy)
- Gastric Bypass (Roux-en-Y)—considered the "Gold Standard" of Bariatric Surgery
- Bilio-Pancreatic Duodenal Switch—rare

## Gastric Sleeve

- Usually Laparoscopic
- 2/3 of stomach is removed
- Stomach becomes tube shaped with restriction at the proximal end
- Inner diameter—16 mm
- Monitor for bleeding & leak
    - Leak—monitor for sepsis
    - Bleeding— ↑ HR, ↓ BP, orthostatic hypotension

## Gastric Bypass (Roux-en-Y)

- Laparoscopic or open
- Create a "pouch" at the upper portion of the stomach
- Small intestine anastomosed to "pouch"
- Pouch only holds ~30 mL
- Initial rapid weight loss
- Monitor for bleeding & leak
- Many experience remission from Type 2 diabetes!

## Post-Op concerns

- Monitor for signs of bleeding
    - ↑ HR, ↓ BP
- Monitor for signs of leaking
    - SIRS, signs of sepsis
- High risk for DVT, pulmonary embolism
    - Mobilize as soon as possible!
- Monitor for hypoglycemia
- Small, frequent, usually liquid or soft meals for 1st week
    - Protein based
- Long term:
    - Dumping syndrome
    - Vitamin deficiencies
    - Lactose intolerance

You can do it!

# Hematology & Immunology Review

## AACN Test Plan for the Hematology & Immunology portion of the PCCN® Exam

- Anemia
- Coagulopathies: medication-induced (i.e., Coumadin, platelet inhibitors, heparin [HIT])

# Anemia

## Who's at Risk?

- Anyone in the ICU > 7 days
- Defined Hgb < 12 g/dL for females & < 13.5 for males
  - Source: American Society of Hematology
- Reasons for anemia:
  - Bleeding (no duh!)
  - Frequent phlebotomy
  - Systemic inflammation
  - ↓ RBC production
  - Iron &/or vitamin $B_{12}$ deficiency
  - Chronic illness
- RBC production is regulated by erythropoietin
- Transfusion threshold.... It depends!!!
- Generally hemoglobin < 7 g/dL, Hematocrit < 21% if the patient is stable
  - Hint: Hemoglobin level multiplied by 3 gives you a hematocrit level
  - If a patient is actively bleeding, don't wait until the Hct is < 21 to transfuse!
  - In actively bleeding patients the transfusion threshold is much higher!

### In general...

- Anemia is tolerated as long as intravascular volume is adequate
- Hemoglobin & hematocrit tell you very little about oxygen utilization!
- All they tell you is how many cells the patient has

## WBCs—Normal 5K – 10K/mm$^3$

### Differential:

- **Neutrophils:** Normal is 55 – 70% of total WBCs
  - Primary responder to infection & inflammation
  - Immature neutrophils are called bands (3 – 6% is normal)
  - Neutropenia—decreased number of neutrophils; high risk for infection!
- **Monocytes:** Normal is 2 – 8% of total WBCs
  - Big phagocytes that mature into macrophages
  - Scavengers of bacteria
- **Lymphocytes:** Normal is 20 – 40% of total WBCs
  - Responsible for adaptive immune response
  - CD4 count is a subset, which is monitored in HIV
- **Eosinophils:** Normal is 1 – 4% of total WBCs
  - ↑ with parasitic infections
  - Will be elevated in allergic response

### Leukocytosis

- Elevation of WBCs (specifically neutrophils) in response to infection or inflammation
- Elevated WBCs are good because they phagocytose bacteria
- Bad because neutrophils release $O_2$ free radicals & excessive cytokines from macrophages

### Leukopenia

- ↓ in the number of WBCs
- See in infection with rapid consumption of WBCs
- Increased risk of infection & immune compromise
- Wash your hands & protect the patient from infection!

### Platelets

- Normal 150,000 – 400,000/uL
- Also called thrombocytes d/t their role in clotting
- ~65% of platelets circulate in blood, ~35% stored in spleen
- Essential for clotting!

# Coagulopathies & Platelet Disorders

- In thrombocytopenia, either there are not enough platelets or the platelet function is impaired
- Life span of a platelet is 10 days
- Any endothelial damage causes platelets to adhere to collagen

### Clot formation process:

Release of calcium →

Activation of Glycoprotein IIb/IIIa receptors on the surface of platelets →

- GP IIb/IIIa receptors bind to fibrinogen to form bridges to other platelets to form clots →
- Calcium activates the coagulation cascade
- End result **→** thrombus

## Thrombocytopenia

- Platelet count < 150,000 /uL
- The body can form platelet plugs until the platelet count is about 100,000 /uL
- Without a structural lesion, we can tolerate platelet count ~ 5,000 /uL as long as there is no major bleeding!
- In ICUs, the incidence of thrombocytopenia is up to 35%
- Causes of thrombocytopenia:
  - Sepsis—Phagocytosis of platelets by macrophages
  - DIC
  - Inflammation
- Symptoms
  - Petechiae
  - Ecchymosis

**Many medications cause impaired platelet functions, here's a short list:**

- » ASA
- » Clopidogrel
- » Prasugrel
- » Pradaxa
- » Glycoprotein inhibitors
- » Ticlidopine
- » Alteplase
- » Heparin
- » Dextran
- » Penicillins
- » Cephalosporins
- » Diphenhydramine
- » Calcium channel blockers
- » Nitroglycerin
- » Nitroprusside
- » Haloperidol
- » Ketorolac

# Immune (Idiopathic) thrombocytopenia purpura (ITP)

- » Autoimmune disorder
- » Antibody mediated destruction of platelets in spleen
- » Platelet counts drop to < 20,000 /uL
- » It is a primary disorder or a secondary disorder due to:
  - Medications
  - Autoimmune disorders (i.e. systemic lupus erythematosus)

**Symptoms:**

- » Petechiae, purpura, epistaxis, splenomegaly

**Treatment:**

- » Corticosteroids
- » IgG-anti-D
- » Immunoglobin IV
- » If refractory:
  - Monoclonal antibody therapy
  - Splenectomy

# Disseminated Intravascular Coagulation (DIC)

The other name for DIC is "Consumptive Coagulopathy"

» Advanced DIC has a mortality up to 80%

» Hypercoagulation secondary to widespread endothelial damage

» Microvascular thrombus formation caused by some predisposing factor like:

- Trauma
- Sepsis/infection
- Obstetric complications

» Release of proinflammtory cytokines → activate the clotting cascade

» Intravascular fibrin formation (micro-emboli)

» Bottom line - use up all the clotting factors, then patients bleed!

## Clinical Presentation

» Tissue & organ ischemia, infarction, organ dysfunction

» Ischemic changes in hands & feet

» Bleeding or oozing from multiple sites in the body

- Petechiae
- Ecchymosis & symmetrical necrosis of limbs
- Purpura Fulminans (blood spots, bruising of skin)
- Gums, mucous membranes, nose
- Oozing from IV sites

## Diagnosis

» Predisposing condition

» Lab values indicate widespread coagulation deficits

» ↓ Platelets; often less than 50,000

» ↑ D-dimer; 1 – 5 mcg/mL

- Advanced > 5 mcg/mL
- Normal is < 0.4 mcg/mL

» ↓ Fibrinogen; < 100 mg/dL

- Normal is 200 – 400 mg/dL

» ↓ Prothrombin Index; 40 – 70, advanced < 40

» ↑ aPTT/PT/INR

» ↑ Fibrin degradation products (FDPs)

### Treatment:

» Treat the cause (i.e. sepsis, trauma, obstetric emergency)

» Supportive

» Volume replacement

» Treat bleeding:

- Platelet transfusions
- Cryoprecipitate
- FFP

# Heparin Induced Thrombocytopenia (HIT)

» Platelet count drops by 30-50% from baseline within 5 – 10 days of exposure to heparin

» May develop more quickly if previous exposure to heparin

» Erythematous lesions around SQ Heparin injection sites

» 25% of patients develop systemic reaction

- Fever
- Chills
- Tachypnea
- Tachycardia
- Generally not associated with bleeding

» **Major Complication: Thrombosis

- Up to 75% of cases may develop systemic thrombosis
- DVT
- MI
- Stroke
- Pulmonary embolism
- Arterial thrombosis to limbs
- Skin necrosis
- End organ damage
- Death

» Risk is greater with unfractionated heparin (UFH)

» Even low doses & heparin flushes

» Don’t forget: heparin coated catheters

## Diagnosis of HIT:

- Clinical exposure to heparin
- Thrombocytopenia
- Symptomatic thrombosis
- IgG antibodies to heparin
  - Platelet factor 4 antibody test
  - IgG with Relex to Serotonin Release Assay
- Clinical picture + assay for diagnosis
- Type I HIT
  - Non-immune mediated
- Type 2 HIT
  - Immune-mediated disorder that typically occurs 4 - 10 days after Heparin exposure
  - Life & limb threatening thrombotic complications

## Treatment of HIT:

- Discontinue all forms of heparin!!!

**Anticoagulation using Direct Thrombin Inhibitors (DTIs):**

- Bivalirudin
  - Initial: 0.15 - 0.2 mg/kg/hr IV
  - Adjust to aPTT 1.5 - 2.5 times baseline value
  - Renal adjustments are necessary
- Argatroban
  - Cleared by the liver
  - 2 mcg/kg/min – Max 10 mcg/kg/min
  - PTT 1.5 – 3 x baseline value, not to exceed 100 seconds
- Long term anticoagulation with Coumadin
  - HOWEVER, do not use during the active phase of HIT
  - Increased risk of limb gangrene
- Heparin antibodies may last > 100 days after exposure
- Do not reintroduce heparin as long as antibodies persist!

# Commonly used anticoagulants

## Coumadin (warfarin)

» Acts on extrinsic & common coagulation pathways

» Monitor PT/INR

- Normal PT = 11 - 13.5 sec
- Normal INR = 0.8 - 1.1

» Therapeutic goal INR 2 – 3x baseline

- DVT prophylaxis
- PE prophylaxis/treatment
- Atrial fibrillation

» Therapeutic goal INR 2.5 – 3.5x baseline

- Mechanical prosthetic valves

» To reverse warfarin:

- Vitamin K (phytonadione) 2.5 – 5 mg PO
- 1 – 2.5 mg IV SLOWLY over an hour
- Will see INR drop within 8 – 12 hours

» Serious or life threatening bleeding

- Vitamin K 10 mg IV SLOWLY—never give IV push!
- Fresh Frozen Plasma (FFP)
- Prothrombin Complex Concentrate (PCC)
    - K-Centra
    - Often used with Vitamin K
- NovoSeven—recombinant factor seven

## Heparin (unfractionated)

» Acts on intrinsic & common coagulation pathways

» Monitor aPTT

- Normal 25 – 38 seconds
- Can also monitor Factor Xa levels

» For procedural sheath removal, can also monitor ACT

- Therapeutic ACT 300 – 350 seconds
- Discontinue sheath when ACT < 150 seconds

» Heparin reversal: Protamine sulfate

### Protamine sulfate for anticoagulation reversal

- Heparin reversal: 1 – 1.5 mg of Protamine per 100 units of Heparin
  - Do not exceed 50 mg Protamine IV
- Dalteparin reversal: 1 mg of Protamine per 100 units of Dalteparin administered
- Enoxaparin reversal: 1 mg of Protamine per 1 mg of enoxaparin if enoxaparin given within 8 hours
- Adverse effects of Protamine:
  - Hypotension
  - Nausea/vomiting
  - Anaphylaxis
  - Flushing
  - May interact w/NPH insulin, PCN or Cephalosporins
  - Anaphylaxis
    - Fish allergies
    - Protamine comes from salmon sperm

## Low Molecular Weight Heparin vs. Unfractionated Heparin

### Benefits of LMWH:

- Less incidence of HIT
- No need to monitor aPTT
- Longer half-life
  - 4 – 6 hours vs. 1 – 2 hours with UFH
- More predictable d/t bioavailability
  - 90% bioavailable vs. 30% with UFH

### Direct Oral Anticoagulation (DOACs)—mostly FYI

- Pradaxa (dabigatran)
  - Used for non-valvular atrial fibrillation, VTE prophylaxis
  - Half-life 12 – 14 hours
  - Praxbind is the reversal agent for bleeding
  - Not used as much
- Xarelto (rivaroxaban)—Direct Factor Xa Inhibitor
  - Used for non-valvular afib, VTE prevention
  - Reversal: Andexxa

- Savaysa, Lixiana (edoxaban)—Direct Factor Xa Inhibitor
  - Used for VTE prophylaxis after ortho surgery, stroke prevention
- Eliquis (apixiban)—Direct Factor Xa Inhibitor
  - Used to prevent venous thromboembolic events
  - Reversal: Andexxa
- Bevyxxa (betrixaban)
  - Direct Factor Xa Inhibitor
  - Venous thromboembolic events, DVT/PE (hospitalized patients)
  - 1-month post discharge (only med with this indication - enoxaparin)
- Other Reversal Notes:
  - If ingested in < 2 hours, activated charcoal
  - Otherwise, control bleeding

# Blood Products

- Whole blood is rarely used, although it's currently being studied in hemorrhaging patients
- It is spun down via centrifuge to:
  - Erythrocytes & plasma
- PRBCs
  - 200 mLs of cells
  - 50 – 100 mLs of CPD & plasma
- Leukocyte-reduced PRBCs often given, but especially if:
  - History of febrile hemolytic transfusion reactions
  - 30% of leukocytes still remain even if leuko-reduced
  - Many blood banks are leuko-reducing PRBCs
- Washed RBCs
  - Reduce leukocytes & plasma
  - Reduces reactions from plasma proteins
- The universal donor is O Negative
- Universal recipient is AB
- Only use 0.9% saline with transfusions...why not Lactated Ringers?
  - LR contains calcium that can promote clotting!!!

## Platelet Transfusions

» When whole blood is donated, platelets get separated with leukocytes
- Increased incidence of fever with platelet transfusion d/t leukocytes

» Banked platelets are usually pooled

» Store banked platelets up to 7 days

» Viability decreases after 3 days

» When a pooled unit of platelets is transfused:
- 30,000/uL rise
- See increase 1 hour after transfusion, lasts up to 8 days

» If not seeing an increase in the platelet count with a transfusion consider:
- Leukocyte reduced transfusion
- ABO compatibility

## PRBCs

» Stored at 4˚C – 21 day shelf life

» CPD preservative
- **C**itrate
  - ▹ Binds to calcium—anticoagulant
  - ▹ Monitor calcium levels when transfusing PRBCs. They can get hypocalcemic!
  - ▹ Patient will need 500 mg – 1 gram of $Ca^{++}$ for every 3 – 4 units of PRBCs
- **P**hosphate
  - ▹ Slows breakdown of 2,3-DPG; banked blood low in 2,3-DPG
  - ▹ 2,3 DPG encourages unloading between $O_2$ & hemoglobin
- **D**extrose
  - ▹ Fuel source for blood cells

» Anticipate calcium replacement when PRBCs are administered!

## Hemolytic Reactions

» Usually human error

» Can also be ABO compatibility

» It only takes about 5 mLs to see a reaction

» Signs:
  - Fever
  - Tachycardia or bradycardia
  - Dyspnea
  - Chest pain
  - Low back pain
  - Hypotension
  - Blood in urine

**Treatment:**

» Stop the transfusion immediately!!!
  - Morbidity & mortality is r/t the amount of blood received

» Monitor vital signs

» Infuse fluids—support BP

» Send unit to the Blood Bank

» Direct & indirect Coomb's Test
  - Positive if there is a hemolytic reaction

You can do it!

# Multi-System Review

## AACN Test Plan for the Multi-System portion of the PCCN® Exam

- Musculoskeletal
  - Immobility, falls, gait disorders
- Healthcare acquired infections (CAUTI, CLABSI, SSI)
  - Infectious disease
- Palliative care
- End-of-life (comfort care measures, hospice)
- Bariatric complications
- Infectious diseases
  - Influenza, multidrug resistant organisms
- Pain
- Sepsis continuum
  - SIRS, Sepsis, Severe Sepsis, Septic Shock
- Shock states
  - Hypovolemic, anaphylactic

### Behavioral/Psychosocial

- Altered mental status
- Delirium
- Dementia
- Psychological disorders
  - Depression, anxiety disorders
- Substance abuse
  - Alcohol withdrawal, chronic alcohol abuse, chronic drug abuse, drug-seeking behavior

# Sepsis

## Early Recognition is Key!!!

- **S**ystemic **I**nflammatory **R**esponse **S**yndrome **(SIRS):**
- ≥ 2 of the following:
  - Temperature > 38.3°C (100.9°F) or < 36°C (96.8°F)
  - Heart rate > 90 bpm
  - RR > 20 bpm or $PaCO_2$ < 32
  - WBC > 12,000 or < 4,000 or > 10% band forms

**If a patient meets SIRS criteria,** do you suspect an infection?

Note: SIRS is also seen in sepsis, burns, trauma, surgery, autoimmune disorders, pancreatitis…so, it is sensitive, but not specific to sepsis!

## Definitions of Sepsis

- Sepsis: 2 SIRS + infection
- Severe Sepsis: Sepsis + Organ dysfunction
- Septic Shock: Severe Sepsis + either: SBP < 90, MAP < 65, or lactate > 4 mmol/L after fluids
  - Severe sepsis + refractory hypotension = Septic shock
  - Abnormal function of > 1 organ = **M**ulti-**O**rgan **D**ysfunction (MODS)

**Common organ involvement:**

- Lungs
  - Monitor for increasing $O_2$ needs or difficulty breathing
- Kidneys
  - Monitor urine output
- Cardiovascular system
  - Monitor signs of decreased C.O., hypotension
- Central nervous system
  - Watch for confusion or LOC changes

### Tissue hypoxia caused by cardiovascular abnormalities

- Vasodilation
- Capillary leak
- Inflammation
- Formation of micro-emboli
- Release of myocardial depressant factor
- Hypercoagulation

### Leads to:

- ↓ intravascular volume
- Tissue edema
- Poor $O_2$ diffusion
- ↓ $O_2$ unloading to the tissues

### Signs of acute organ dysfunction:

- Altered consciousness, confusion, psychosis
- Tachypnea, $PaO_2$ < 70 mm Hg, $SpO_2$ < 90%, $PaO_2$/ $FiO_2$ (P/F ratio) ≤ 300
- ↑ $O_2$ needs
- Jaundice, ↑ LFTs, ↑ bilirubin, ↓ albumin, ↑ PT/INR
- Tachycardia, hypotension
- Oliguria, anuria, ↑ creatinine
- ↓ Platelets, ↓ protein C, ↑ D-dimer
- Hemodynamics of severe sepsis & septic shock ↑ CO, ↓ afterload, ↓ preload (early)

## 3 & 6 Hour Sepsis Bundles (CMS)

### Early detection—1st 3 hours

- Measure lactate level
- Obtain blood cultures ideally prior to administration of antibiotics
- Administer broad spectrum antibiotics
  - Do not delay especially in shock!

» Administer 30 ml/kg crystalloid for hypotension or lactate ≥ 4 mmol/L

- FYI—There's building evidence to use LR or Plasmalyte-A over 0.9% saline
- ↑ Incidence of AKI w/saline

## Critical Care—1st 6 hours

» Apply vasopressors for hypotension that does not respond to fluid resuscitation to maintain MAP ≥ 65 mm Hg

- Norepinephrine infusion
- Vasopressin infusion (2nd line agent)

» For persistent hypotension after initial fluid administration, or if initial lactate was ≥ 4 mmol/L, reassess volume status & tissue perfusion

» Re-measure lactate if initial was elevated

» Dynamic assessment of fluid responsiveness with passive leg raise or fluid challenge

## Lactate

» In sepsis, lactate should be viewed as a marker of tissue perfusion

» Lactate has some prognostic utility

- 0 – 2.5 mmol/L 4.9% mortality
- 2.5 – 4.0 mmol/L 9.0%
- > 4.0 mmol/L 28.4%

» Sustained elevated lactate > 6 hours portends increased mortality

» Mortality increases as lactate levels increase

## Lactate Clearance

» Re-measure lactate after fluids or interventions

» It should decrease; ideally by at least 10% with each intervention

» The goal is to normalize the lactate by improving perfusion

### $ScvO_2$:

- $ScvO_2$ Goal > 70%
  - Surrogate of mixed venous ($SvO_2$)
  - Can measure intermittently via central line or PICC line
  - Draw a sample of blood from the distal port of a central line

### Sepsis key points...

- Early recognition
- In the 1st 3 hours:
  - Labs – Lactate, CBC with differential, cultures
  - Fluids (30 ml/kg to start)
  - Repeat lactate after fluid boluses
  - Antibiotics: Broad spectrum, then narrow
  - Source control
  - Prevent critical care!!!

# Anaphylaxis

- Inflammatory response & hypersensitivity reaction

### Common allergens:

- Contrast dye
- Food
- Antimicrobials
- Insect bites
- Symptoms minutes to hours

### Less serious reactions:

- Flushing
- Erythema
- Rash
- Urticaria
- Diarrhea

## More serious:

- Angioedema
- Laryngeal edema
- Tongue swelling
- Bronchospasm
- Hypotension

## Anaphylaxis treatment:

### 1st Line Treatment: Epinephrine!

- Monitor airway!!!
- Epinephrine 1:1,000 strength
  - Most concentrated
  - 0.3 mg IM
- Blocks the release of inflammatory mediators
- Can also nebulize the epinephrine to treat laryngeal edema
- If taking a beta blocker, can give Glucagon 5 – 15 mcg/min IV continuous infusion

### 2nd Line Treatment: (Histamine blockers)

- Diphenhydramine 25 – 50 mg IV/IM/PO
  - $H_1$ blocker
- Ranitidine 50 mg IV or 150 mg PO or Pepcid (famotidine) 20 mg IV
  - $H_2$ blocker
- Synergistic effect
- Steroids—prevent 2nd phase symptoms
  - Prednisone 50 mg PO or
  - Methylprednisolone 125 mg IV
- If progression to anaphylactic shock:
  - Massive vasodilation with fluid shifts
  - ↓ afterload & preload
  - Volume resuscitation
  - Consider colloids
  - ICU transfer!
- For refractory hypotension:
  - Vasoconstrictors to constrict or "tighten up" the vasculature
    - Epinephrine infusion 2–8 mcg/min
    - Dopamine infusion 5–20 mcg/kg/min
    - Norepinephrine infusion 2 – 8 mcg/min

# Overdoses

## Acetaminophen Overdose:

- Included in over 600 drug preparations
- Leading cause of toxic ingestions & acute liver failure
- Over 1/3 are unintentional
- 80 – 90% metabolized through the liver
- Toxic metabolite accumulates & causes widespread hepatocellular damage

### Risk Assessment:

- Determine ingested dose—amount & time
- Approximately 7.5 to 15 grams can cause toxicity
  - Lower in some patients
- Concomitant use of ETOH increases risk
- Assess plasma acetaminophen levels
  - Measure 4 – 24° after ingestion to predict risk
- If the level falls in the high risk category of the Rumack-Matthew nomogram, risk of hepatotoxicity is ≥ 60%

### 4 Stages of Toxicity:

#### 1st 24 hours after ingestion:

- No or vague symptoms
- No lab value / evidence of injury

#### 24 – 72 hours:

- No or vague symptoms
- ↑ AST—most sensitive
- Precedes hepatic dysfunction

**72 – 96 hours:**

- Progressive hepatic injury
- Peak AST levels
- Encephalopathy
- Coagulopathy
- Renal dysfunction & failure

**3 – 5 days:**

- Start recovery or death

## Treatment:

- Antidote: N-Acetylcysteine (Mucomyst or NAC)
  - Limits accumulation of the metabolite to prevent hepatocellular damage
  - Replenishes glutathione to react with metabolites (NAC)
  - Ideal to start within 24 hours of ingestion
  - IV preferred d/t smell
- Activated charcoal is also an option if used within 4 hours of ingestion

## N-Acetylcysteine (NAC) dosing:

- IV dosing: 150 mg/kg over 15 - 30 min.
  - 50 mg/kg over 4 hrs, then 100 mg/kg over 16 hrs
  - Total: 300 mg/kg over 21 hrs
- PO dosing: 140 mg/kg PO load, then 70 mg/kg Q 4 hours
  - Total: 1330 mg/kg over 72 hrs
  - 17 doses after loading dose
  - Smells like rotten eggs, so may not be tolerated

# Benzodiazepine Overdose:

- 2nd most common overdose in the US
- Usually involves a 2nd respiratory depressant

### Higher risk:

- Advanced age
- Accumulative dosing
- Assess for concomitant use with opioids

### Treatment:

****Antagonist: Flumazenil (Romazicon)**

- IV - 0.2 mg repeated Q 1 – 6 min up to 1 mg
    - Onset: 1 – 2 min
    - Peak: 6 – 10 min
    - Duration: 60 min
- Duration of benzos often last longer than the antidote
- Monitor for re-sedation
- Can do continuous Flumazenil infusion 0.3 – 0.4 mg/hr
- Monitor for benzo withdrawal; can precipitate seizures

## Aspirin (Salicylate) Overdose:

### Diagnosis:

- Clinical presentation
- Anion gap (+ gap)
- ABGs
    - Respiratory alkalosis d/t brain stimulation of respiratory center (medulla)
- Monitor serum salicylate levels
- Acute ingestion of > 150 mg/kg can cause severe toxicity
- Salicylate tablets may form bezoars, prolonging absorption & toxicity
    - Need to know if enteric coated

### Signs:

- Vomiting
- Tinnitus
- Confusion
- Hyperthermia
- Metabolic acidosis
- Irregular breathing patterns
  - Can lead to respiratory alkalosis
- Multiple organ failure

### Treatment:

- Activated charcoal
- Bicarb infusion
- Alkaline diuresis
- IV fluids
- Hemodialysis
- Supportive

## Opioid Overdose:

- Morphine, dilaudid & fentanyl most common in hospitalized patients
- Heroin for street drugs
- Major problem: bradycardia, hypotension & respiratory depression

### Treatment:

#### Antagonist: Naloxone (Narcan)

- Binds to opioid receptors
- Dose: 0.4 mg IV or IM
  - Onset IV: 2 - 3 min, IM 5 - 15 min
  - Repeat in 2 min up to 1 mg
  - Opioid dependency dose 0.1 – 0.2 mg
- Monitor for recurrent respiratory depression
  - For respiratory depression or resp arrest: repeat dosing Q 2 min up to 10 mg
  - Effects last 60 min
  - Can also consider a Naloxone infusion

### Adverse effects of Naloxone:

- Anxiety
- Abdominal cramping
- N/V
- Piloerection

## Beta Blocker Overdose:

- Over 15 FDA approved in the US

### Side effects:

- Bradycardia
- Hypotension
  - d/t vasodilation & renin blockade
- Decreased C.O.
- $B_1$ receptor blockade
- Heart block from prolonged A-V conduction

### Neurotoxicity:

- Lethargy, ↓ LOC, seizures
- Seizures more common with Propranolol

### Antidote: Glucagon

- 3 mg IV initial dose (0.05 mcg/kg)
- 5 mg IV repeated dose (0.07 mcg/kg)
- Continuous infusion 5 mg/hr if needed
- Reverses the $B_1$ blockade
- Mimics + inotropic effects of beta receptor activation
- Atropine may be needed for the bradycardia
  - Give the Glucagon first
  - Prepare to emergently pace

### Side effects of Glucagon:

- N/V
- Mild hyperglycemia
- Hypokalemia
- Hypertension

## Calcium Channel Blocker Overdose:

- Over 10 FDA approved
- Verapamil, nifedipine & diltiazem most common
- $Ca^{++}$ influx into myocardial cells is essential & determines strength of contraction

### Effects:

- Negative inotropic effects (reduces C.O.)
- Negative chronotropic effects (bradycardia)
- Prolonged AV conduction
- Vasodilation
- Bronchial dilation

### Neuro effects:

- Lethargy
- ↓ LOC
- Generalized seizures
- Hyperglycemia (inhibits insulin release)

### Treatment:

- Calcium!!!
- Calcium chloride 10% IV
  - 1 amp = 1.36 mEq/ml
  - Prevent blockade – 3 ml
  - Reverse blockade – 10 ml/13.6 mEq
- Calcium gluconate 10% IV
  - 1 amp = 0.46 mEq/ml
  - Prevent blockade – 10 ml
  - Reverse blockade – 30 ml/13.8 mEq

- Can use continuous IV since effects are so short lived (10 – 15 min)
  - 0.3 – 0.7 mEq/kg/hr
- Atropine 0.5 – 1.0 mg IV
  - Reverse bradycardia
  - Give $Ca^{++}$ first!!!
  - Atropine is enhanced by calcium administration
- If continued hypotension, use catecholamine infusion:
  - Epinephrine, norepinephrine or dopamine

## Tricyclic Antidepressant (TCA) Overdose

### Examples:

- Amitriptyline (Elavil)
- Nortriptyline (Pamelor)

### Signs:

- Hyperthermia
- Hypotension
  - Fluids & norepinephrine
- Tachycardia
  - Get a 12 Lead ECG
  - Wide QRS – give sodium bicarb
  - ***Prolonged QTc
  - Anti-arrhythmics do not help; may actually make it worse!
- Confusion
- Seizures
  - Benzos!
- Dilated pupils
- Cardiac Arrest

### Treatment:

- Activated charcoal
- Sodium Bicarbonate if having arrythmias
- Magnesium IV

## Cocaine Toxicity

- Alpha & Beta stimulant
- Risk of MI & stroke

### Symptoms:

- Tachycardia
- Hypertension
- Fever
- Coronary spasm/MI

### Treatment:

- Benzodiazepines
  - Increases the action of GABA & depresses the CNS
- Vasodilators if hypertensive
- Avoid beta blockers!
  - Leave unopposed alpha receptor stimulation

# ETOH Withdrawal

- Potentially life threatening
- Sudden cessation of alcohol intake or reduced consumption
- Symptoms can start as early as 2 hours & continue for weeks
- ~80% of AWS are mild requiring only symptom management
- Abrupt cessation leads to brain hyperexcitability
- Alcohol/Ethanol leads to:
  - GABA inhibition
  - ETOH-mediated inhibition of NMDA receptors
  - Stimulates effects of glutamate
  - Excess norepinephrine (NE) d/t desensitization of alpha-2 receptors

## Symptoms of withdrawal:

- » Tachycardia
- » Tachypnea
- » Tremors
  - Can involve tongue & upper extremities
- » Anxiety
- » Irritation
- » Sweating
- » Adrenergic Stress
- » Withdrawal seizures
  - Peak in 12 – 48 hours after cessation of ETOH
  - Grand mal seizures occur in 5 – 15% of AWS
  - In general, the more ETOH consumed, the greater the risk of seizures
- » DTs—delirium tremens

## Clinical Institute Withdrawal Assessment Scale (CIWA) assesses:

- » Nausea & vomiting
- » Paroxysmal sweating
- » Agitation
- » Visual disturbances
- » Tremor
- » Tactile disturbances
- » Headache
- » Auditory disturbances
- » Orientation/clouding sensorium

## Scoring:

- » < 8: No medications needed
- » 9 – 14: Optional medications
- » 15 – 19: Give medication
- » 20: High risk for complications

## Treatment of DTs

### Pharmacologic:

- Benzodiazepines
  - Lorazepam or Valium
  - Current standard of care
  - Monitor for delirium
- Librium
- Phenobarbital
  - Anti-convulsant properties
- Dexmetomidine (Precedex)
  - Alpha - 2 agonist
  - Monitor for bradycardia
- Low dose anti-psychotics
  - Haldol
  - Quetiapine (Seroquel)
  - Monitor for prolonged QTc interval
- IV fluids
- Electrolyte imbalance ($Mg^{++}$)
- Thiamine ($B_1$)
- Anti-seizure medications
  - Prophylactic if previous seizures from withdrawal
  - Carbamazepine
  - Valproic Acid (VPA)
  - Gabapentin
  - Pregabalin

### Nursing:

- Safety
- Quiet environment
- Airway
- Seizure precautions
- Cardiac monitoring
- Monitor QTc if giving anti-psychotics
- In general, elderly at higher risk

# Delirium

- » Acute brain dysfunction
- » 3 Key characteristics:
  - Inattention
  - Confusion
  - Disorganized thinking
- » Can wax & wane
- » Hyperactive & hypoactive
  - Hypoactive is more common

## Who is at risk?

- » Hospitalized patients
- » Elderly
- » Stroke, CNS issues
- » Sepsis
- » Sleep deprived
- » Electrolyte imbalances
- » Dehydration
- » Memory impaired
- » Severe burns or trauma
- » Let's be honest…everyone!

## Monitoring for delirium

- » Confusion Assessment Method (CAM)
- » Most validated tool & widely used
- » Assess for fluctuation in neuro status from baseline
- » Assess RASS (or sedation level)

## PADIS Guidelines

Guidelines to give direction on how to prevent & manage delirium

**P** = **Pain**

**A** = **Agitation**

**D** = **Delirium**

**I** = **Immobility**

**S** = **Sleep disturbances**

### Pain

- Treat pain first!!!
- Use a behavioral pain assessment scale
- Ask the right questions
- Do not use sedatives to treat pain
- Pre-emptive pain plan for:
    - Treatments
    - Mobility
    - Dressing changes

### Agitation

- Minimize sedation
- Avoid benzodiazepines
    - Unless ETOH withdrawal
- Consider non-benzodiazepines for sedation if needed
    - Dexmetomidine (Precedex)
- Don't overuse sedation; "light" sedation
    - RASS—1 to 0 should be the goal
- Daily interruption in sedation (wake patient up)
- Determine sedation goal
- Remove any unnecessary lines or tubes
- Consider non-pharmacologic interventions

## Delirium

- Prevent it!!!
- Monitor for it!!!
- Identify who is at risk
- If the patient develops delirium:
  - Identify reversible causes:

    **T** = Toxins

    **H** = Hypoxemia

    **I** = Infection

    **N** = Non-pharmacologic interventions

    **K** = $K^+$ (electrolyte imbalances—$Na^+$ is a big one!)
  - Avoid benzodiazepines
  - Dexmetomidine (Precedex) associated with lower delirium risk vs. benzo
- Review the medication list—eliminate any meds not necessary
- Pharmacist consult

## General prevention considerations:

- Glasses & hearing aids on the patient!
- Day/night orientation
- Method of communicating if barrier
- Frequent reorientation
- Mobility!
- Minimize or avoid benzo use
- Board in room with place & date
- Clock in view
- Noise control
- Promote sleep
- Cluster care activities

# Rhabdomyolysis

- Muscle injury release myoglobin into the blood
- Large protein molecules can lead to acute kidney injury
- Most cases are reversible if promptly treated

## Causes:

- Trauma, crush injuries
- Extreme temps
- Exercise
- Immobilization
- Electrical shock injury
- Cocaine, meth, ETOH
- Statins (rare)

## Diagnostics:

- CPK, myoglobin
- Urine myoglobin
- Electrolytes
- BUN & creatinine

## Symptoms:

- Dark, brown or reddish colored urine
- Muscle pain
- Muscle weakness
    - ~50% have no muscle symptoms
- Abdominal pain
- Fever
- N/V

## Complications:

- Acute kidney injury (AKI) from myoglobinuria
- Hyperkalemia
- Metabolic acidosis

**Treatment:**

- IV fluids
- Dialysis if needed
- Monitor for compartment syndrome of the extremities
- Fasciotomy if warranted

# Carbon Monoxide Poisoning

- Replaces oxygen on hemoglobin cells

**Symptoms:**

- Hypoxia
- Headache
- Altered LOC
- Seizures

**Treatment:**

- Administer oxygen
- Mechanical ventilation if needed
- Hyperbaric oxygen therapy

# Skin

- Is the largest organ in the body
- High risk areas:
    - Coccyx, buttocks, scalp, heels
- Consults to PT & Nutrition are helpful

## Staging pressure injury

**(I would recommend doing a quick review of this while studying!)**

Source: https://npuap.org/page/PressureInjuryStages

### Stage 1 Pressure Injury:

» Non-blanchable erythema of intact skin Intact skin with a localized area of non-blanchable erythema, which may appear differently in darkly pigmented skin

» Presence of blanchable erythema or changes in sensation, temperature, or firmness may precede visual changes

» Color changes do not include purple or maroon discoloration; these may indicate deep tissue pressure injury

### Stage 2 Pressure Injury:

» Partial-thickness skin loss with exposed dermis

» The wound bed is viable, pink or red, moist, & may also present as an intact or ruptured serum-filled blister

» Adipose (fat) is not visible & deeper tissues are not visible

» Granulation tissue, slough & eschar are not present

» These injuries commonly result from adverse microclimate & shear in the skin over the pelvis & shear in the heel

» This stage should not be used to describe moisture associated skin damage (MASD) including incontinence associated dermatitis (IAD), intertriginous dermatitis (ITD), medical adhesive related skin injury (MARSI), or traumatic wounds (skin tears, burns, abrasions)

## Stage 3 Pressure Injury:

- Full-thickness loss of skin, in which adipose (fat) is visible in the ulcer & granulation tissue & epibole (rolled wound edges) are often present
- Slough and/or eschar may be visible
- The depth of tissue damage varies by anatomical location; areas of significant adiposity can develop deep wounds
- Undermining & tunneling may occur
- Fascia, muscle, tendon, ligament, cartilage and/or bone are not exposed
- If slough or eschar obscures the extent of tissue loss this is an Unstageable Pressure Injury

## Stage 4 Pressure Injury:

- Full-thickness skin & tissue loss with exposed or directly palpable fascia, muscle, tendon, ligament, cartilage or bone in the ulcer
- Slough and/or eschar may be visible
- Epibole (rolled edges), undermining and/or tunneling often occur
- Depth varies by anatomical location
- If slough or eschar obscures the extent of tissue loss this is an Unstageable Pressure Injury

## Unstageable Pressure Injury:

- Obscured full-thickness skin & tissue loss in which the extent of tissue damage within the ulcer cannot be confirmed because it is obscured by slough or eschar
- If slough or eschar is removed, a Stage 3 or Stage 4 pressure injury will be revealed
- Stable eschar (i.e. dry, adherent, intact without erythema or fluctuance) on the heel or ischemic limb should not be softened or removed

**Deep Tissue Pressure Injury:**

- Persistent non-blanchable deep red, maroon or purple discoloration Intact or non-intact skin with localized area of persistent non-blanchable deep red, maroon, purple discoloration or epidermal separation revealing a dark wound bed or blood-filled blister
- Pain & temperature change often precede skin color changes
- Discoloration may appear differently in darkly pigmented skin
- This injury results from intense and/or prolonged pressure & shear forces at the bone-muscle interface
- The wound may evolve rapidly to reveal the actual extent of tissue injury, or may resolve without tissue loss
- If necrotic tissue, subcutaneous tissue, granulation tissue, fascia, muscle or other underlying structures are visible, this indicates a full thickness pressure injury (Unstageable, Stage 3 or Stage 4)
- Do not use DTPI to describe vascular, traumatic, neuropathic, or dermatologic conditions

# Shock States

**Know how the body responds in different states of shock!**

| Shock State | HR | BP | CO | Preload | Afterload |
|---|---|---|---|---|---|
| Hypovolemic Shock | ↑ | ↓ | ↓ | ↓ | ↑ |
| Cardiogenic Shock | ↑ | ↓ | ↓ | ↑ | ↑ |
| Septic Shock | ↑/= | ↓ | ↑ | ↓ | ↓ |
| Anaphylactic Shock | ↑ | ↓ | ↓ | ↓ | ↓ |

# Neurology Review

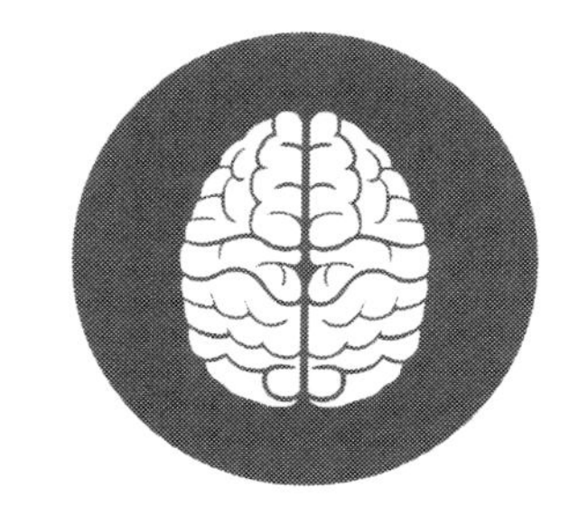

## AACN Test Plan for the Neurology portion of the PCCN® Exam

- Encephalopathy
  - Hypoxic-ischemic, metabolic, infectious, hepatic
- Seizure Disorders
- Stroke
  - Ischemic/embolic, hemorrhagic, transient ischemic attack – TIA

# Brain anatomy & function

- Frontal lobe:
  - Personality, motor function, motor speech, morals, emotions, judgment
- Parietal lobe:
  - Sensation, pain interpretation, temperature, pressure
- Temporal lobe:
  - Auditory & speech
- Occipital lobe:
  - Visual
- Cerebellum:
  - Coordination of muscle movement & tone, coordination, equilibrium
- Brain Stem:
  - Messages between the brain & body
  - Basic functions—breathing, HR & BP control, swallow, awakeness

## The Brain:

- Brain compartment is comprised of:
  - 80% Tissue
  - 10% CSF
  - 10% Blood
- Two lateral ventricles
- Third & Fourth Ventricles
- Foramen of Monro:
  - Conduit of CSF flow from the lateral ventricles to the third ventricle

## Cerebral Spinal Fluid (CSF)

- Clear, colorless
- Large amount of $Na^+$, $Cl^-$, glucose & some protein
- Cushions & protects the brain & spinal cord
- 500 ml produced per day

### Monro-Kellie Doctrine:

- Balance of tissue, CSF & blood to create an equilibrium
- ↑ in one area must result in a ↓ in another
- If not, the intracranial pressure (ICP) will increase!
  - Compression of venous blood
  - Displacement of CSF
  - Blood flow is maintained by cerebral auto-regulation

### Causes of Intracranial Hypertension:

- Trauma—TBI
- Intracranial Hemorrhage
- Hydrocephalus
- Cerebral edema
- Stroke
- Brain tumors
- Hypoxic-ischemic brain injury (cardiac arrest)
- Brain infections/abscess
- Fever
- Seizures

### External Causes of Intracranial Hypertension:

- Suctioning
- Position changes
- Nursing care
- Positive End-Expiratory Pressure (PEEP)—i.e. Bi-Pap
- Increased stimuli

## Neuro Assessment

- Level of consciousness
- Mentation: Are there changes? Even slight?
- Pupillary response: Equal & reactive?
- Motor skills: Equal on both sides?
  - Against resistance?

- » Sensory deficits?
  - Test with light touch/pinprick
- » Vision or speech deficits?
- » Cranial Nerve Assessment
- » Glasgow Coma Scale measures:
  - Best eye response
  - Best verbal response
  - Best motor response

## Signs of Increased Intracranial Pressure (ICP)

- » **Change in LOC
- » Headache
- » Nausea/vomiting
  - Can progress to projectile
- » Lethargy
- » Irritability
- » Slow decision making

## Late changes:

- » Pupillary changes
- » Dilation in one eye
- » Seizures
- » Posturing
- » Can progress to coma

### Methods of monitoring ICP

- » Intra-ventricular catheter
  - Used to drain excessive CSF & intermittently monitor ICP
- » Intraparenchymal (ICU)
  - Monitor pressure only
  - Commonly referred to as a "bolt"

# Managing increased ICP

## First Tier Interventions:

» Patient positioning
- Manage venous drainage

» Prevent compression of jugular veins

» HOB 30 – 45 degrees

» Good head alignment—keep midline

» Straighten legs

» ↓ stimuli

» Analgesics—assess for pain

» Normothermia
- Fever associated with worse outcomes

## Second Tier Interventions:

» Mannitol 20% - Osmotic diuretic
- 0.25 to 1 gram/kg IV bolus
- ICP ↓ within 5 – 10 min
- Maximum effect in 1 hour
- Use filter!
- May repeat q 1 – 4 hours
- Monitor Osmolality, $Na^+$ & $K^+$ levels

» Hypertonic Saline (Usually 3%)
- Continuous infusion
- Monitor osmolality & $Na^+$ levels

» Loop Diuretics
- ↓ intracranial blood volume

» Considerations for all:
- Monitor serum osmo & fluid status
- OSMO no higher than 320 mOsm/L
  - Or patient specific goal
- Monitor for signs of rebound ↑ in ICP
- Potassium levels
  - Can get hypokalemic from treatment

# Stroke

- 5th leading cause of death in the US
- Leading cause of disability
- Hypertension is the biggest risk factor
  - Atrial fibrilation
  - Patent foramen ovale
- Dysphagia is common & can lead to aspiration pneumonia
- 2 Types:
- Ischemic/embolic ~ 85%
  - May present with transient ischemic attack (TIA)
    - Warning sign of stroke
    - Blood supply to brain tissue briefly halting
- Hemorrhagic ~ 15%

## AHA Stroke Guidelines

- 1 hour goals:
  - Complete National Institute of Health Stroke Scale (NIHSS) Assessment
  - CT Scan without contrast
  - Assess glucose level
  - Treat with fibrinolytic therapy (if appropriate)
  - Large vessel occlusions (LVO) benefit from thrombectomy

## NIH Stroke Scale assesses:

- LOC
- Eye deviation (CN III, VI, VIII)
- Visual field loss (hemianopia)
- Facial palsy
- Motor arms (drift)
- Motor legs
- Limb ataxia
- Sensory
- Language
- Dysarthria
- Extinction & inattention
- Note: Higher score consistent with more severe stroke
  - Scores 0 - 42
  - Not a diagnostic tool

### Diagnostics:

- CT scan <u>without</u> contrast within 20 minutes of arrival
  - R/O hemorrhage
  - Should be interpreted within 45 min
  - Might see hypodensity in ischemic area with embolic stroke
- CT perfusion or MRI perfusion
  - Measures infarct core or penumbra

## Treatment: rtPA

### rtPA Considerations:

- "Door to needle" time = 1 hour
- Symptom onset window = extended 4.5 hour window, but shortened to 3 hours if:
  - Age > 80
  - Taking oral anticoagulation regardless of the INR
  - History of stroke & diabetes
  - Baseline NIHSS score > 25
- Baseline labs/tests:
  - Glucose is the only requirement
  - CBC, coags, chemistry, troponin, 12 lead ECG are ideal
- **Control BP prior to administration!!**
  - Goal SBP < 185, DBP < 110
- Dosing rtPA: 0.9 mg/kg IV, maximum of 90 mg
  - 10% of dose given over the 1st minute
  - The remaining infused over 1 hour

### Other medication tips:

- If the patient received therapeutic doses of LMWH in the previous 24 hours, avoid rtPA
  - This does NOT include prophylactic doses!

- Abciximab (Reopro) should NOT be administered concomitantly
- Aspirin 325 mg should be given within 24 - 48 hours of stroke onset
- Do not provide other anticoagulation therapy within 24 hours of rtPA
- Begin statin therapy**
  - Restart statins if they were previously taking them

## BP reduction strategies:

- **Carefully** lower the BP
- Avoid swings in BP!
- BP goal:
  - < 185/110 before alteplase is administered!
- Which medications should be used?
  - Labetalol 10 – 20 mg IV over 1 – 2 min, repeat
  - Nicardipine 5 mg/hour IV, titrate up to 15 mg/hour max
  - Clevidipine 1 – 2 mg/hour, max 21 mg/hour
  - Hydralazine IV
  - Enalaprilat

## Complications of rtPA include conversion to hemorrhage

- Conversion to ICH risk ~ 6%
  - Some sources cite lower rates
- Symptoms:
  - Deteriorating neuro exam
  - Headache
  - Nausea/vomiting
  - Acute hypertension
- Actions:
  - Prepare for STAT head CT scan
  - Stat coags, fibrinogen, CBC
- Prepare to transfuse if appropriate:
  - Platelets
  - Cryoprecipitate
    - Contains fibrinogen & clotting factors
  - Tranexamic acid (TXA)
    - Antifibrinolytic
  - FFP
    - Caution with the volume associated with administration!

## Endovascular therapies for ischemic stroke:

- Newer evidence to support endovascular procedures for large vessel occlusion
- Should receive rtPA regardless
- May be reasonable in patients with a contraindication to IV fibrinolysis
- Intra-arterial rtPA may also be considered

## Stroke care components:

- Cardiac monitoring
  - Atrial fibrillation & cardiac arrhythmias are common causes of stroke
  - TEE to assess for thrombus
    - Left atrium & appendage often the culprit
- Echocardigram
  - Assess for Atrial Septal Defect (ASD) or Patent Foramen Ovale (PFO) as cause of stroke
  - Bubble study
- Restart anti-hypertensives after 24 hours
  - Should have specific BP targets!
  - Higher target if no rtPA
- Airway support
  - Ventilatory assistance if needed
  - Apply $O_2$ if sats are < 94%
  - Aspiration risk
- Avoid fever!!! (temp > 37.5˚C)
  - Antipyretic therapy
  - Fever = ↑ morbidity & mortality
- Treat hypovolemia
- Treat hypoglycemia (< 70 mg/dL)
  - Goal: 140 - 180
  - Hyperglycemia is a common neuroendocrine stress response
  - Worse outcomes if hyper or hypoglycemic
- DVT prophylaxis
  - Prophylactic anticoagulation &/or SCDs
  - Early mobilization
- NPO until swallow evaluation
  - Nurse-driven swallow screen
  - If unable to take solids, consider placing a feeding tube
  - If > 2 weeks, consider PEG
- Avoid in-dwelling urinary catheters
  - High risk of UTIs specifically in the neuro population

### Nursing considerations for stroke care:

- Frequent neuro checks
  - Monitor for signs of increased ICP
  - Placement of a Ventriculostomy drain if hydrocephalus develops
- Monitor for bleeding
  - Conversion of embolic to hemorrhagic stroke
- Corticosteroids are not routinely recommended
- Monitor for seizures
  - Acute ischemic stroke is one of the highest causes of epilepsy in the elderly
  - Routine prophylaxis is not indicated

### Therapies to consider for stroke:

- Physical Therapy
- Occupational Therapy
- Speech
- Long term placement if ongoing disability
- Palliative Care if appropriate
- Depression is common

# Carotid Stenosis

### Clinical presentation:

- TIAs, visual Δ's
- Memory loss
- Vertigo, syncope
- Carotid bruit or thrill

### Treatment:

- Antiplatelet aggregation (ASA, Plavix)
- BP control
  - Specific patient targets should be established
  - Do not want to lower too much
- Carotid Endarterectomy
- Carotid Stenting
- Balloon angioplasty (not done as much)

### Carotid Endarterectomy:

- Post-op: Monitor for bleeding/hematoma
- Close airway monitoring d/t location of incision swelling
- Regular neuro assessments post-op
- Cranial nerve assessment:
  - VII: Smile
  - IX/X: Swallow, gag, speech
  - XI: Shrug shoulders
  - XII: Stick out tongue

# Transient Ischemic Attacks (TIAs)

- "Mini stroke"
- Similar symptoms to stroke
- Temporary disruption in blood flow
- Resolves & symptoms usually go away within 24 hours
- Doesn't cause permanent damage to brain cells
- Precursor to a stroke
- Plan for carotid ultrasound

# Hemorrhagic Stroke

### Causes:

- Subarachnoid Hemorrhage (SAH)
  - Aneurysm, AV Malformation
- Intracranial Hemorrhage (ICH)
  - Spontaneous rupture of a blood vessel
    - Chronic HTN
- Brain tumor bleed
- Uncontrolled anticoagulation
- Recreational drugs
- Hemorrhagic conversion after rtPA

### Who's at risk?

- Hypertension—the big one!
- Diabetes
- Atrial fibrillation
  - Due to anticoagulation

- Smokers
- Geriatric population
- Trauma

### Symptoms:

- Abrupt & rapid onset
- Severe headache
- Nuchal rigidity
- Hemiparesis
- Posturing
- Stupor, coma

****Severity depends on the location & size of the bleed**

### Treatment:

- Consider BP reduction if:
  - SBP > 200 or MAP > 150
  - More aggressive if signs of increased ICP & SBP > 180
- Airway support
- Monitor for seizures
- Nursing care same as ischemic stroke
- Supportive treatment

# Aneurysms

- Most occur in the anterior arteries of the Circle of Willis
- Rupture most likely when > 8 – 10 mm
- Congenital, vessel weakness or unknown
- Bleed into subarachnoid space
  - CSF will be bloody

### Risk factors:

- Family history
- Congenital
- HTN
- Smokers
- Polycystic kidney disease (chronic hypertension)

## Diagnosis:

- CT Scan WITHOUT contrast

## Symptoms:

- Many are asymptomatic until they bleed/rupture
- Symptoms & prognosis depend on the area & size of bleed
- Sudden headache
- "Worst headache of my life"
- Nausea/vomiting
- Photophobia
- Diplopia
- Nuchal rigidity
- Kernig's sign and/or Brudzinski's sign
  - Indicates meningeal irritation
- Seizures
- Decreased LOC, may progress to coma

## Treatment:

- BP control
  - In general, keep SBP 140 - 180 mm Hg, much lower before securement!
  - Needs to be patient specific target
  - Higher targets after securement
- Monitor for re-bleed
- Days 4 – 14 monitor for cerebral artery vasospasm
  - Transcranial Doppler to monitor
  - High velocities indicative of spasm
  - Start prophylactic calcium channel blocker to prevent spasm
    - Nimotop (Nimodipine) most commonly used
    - Administered for about 1 month

## Post bleed/intervention, monitor for signs of:

- Increased ICP
- Cerebral edema
- Hydrocephalus

### Interventions:

- » Surgical & endovascular securement

## Arterial-Venous Malformation (AVM)

- » Entanglement of blood vessels
- » Concern with bleed or rupture
- » Surgical and/or endovascular treatment
- » Often congenital

## Symptoms—all strokes

### Right cerebral hemisphere:

- » Left sided motor symptoms
- » Respond well to verbal cues
- » Can understand language
- » Assists with cognition (thinking)
- » Difficulty starting a conversation
- » Rambling speech
- » Issues with problem solving

### Left cerebral hemisphere:

- » Right sided motor symptoms
- » Aphasia
- » Expressive aphasia
    - Inability to express verbally in an understandable manner
- » Receptive aphasia
    - Inability to understand spoken words
- » Dyslexia
- » Acalculia
    - Difficulty performing simple math
- » Right & left disorientation
- » May respond well to pictures
- » Memory loss
- » Emotionally labile

# Detailed Stroke Symptoms

## Weakness & Hemiparesis

- » Neurons cross either in the:
  - Spinal cord
  - Brainstem
  - Brain
- » Weakness or paralysis on opposite side of body
- » Right-sided weakness may likely have aphasia
- » Left-sided weakness may see neglect
- » Often, look toward the stroke

## Speech

- » 40% of stroke patients develop language problems post stroke
- » Broca's area – frontal lobe of the brain
  - Fluid speech production
  - Slow, poorly articulated speech
- » Wernicke's area
  - Understanding
  - Producing meaningful speech
- » Most people are left hemisphere dominant (right-handed) = aphasia!
- » Expressive aphasia
  - Difficulty converting thoughts to language
- » Receptive aphasia
  - Difficulty understanding written & verbal language
  - Can the patient follow commands?
  - Can likely understand non-verbal language

## Middle cerebral artery (MCA)

- » Most common strokes
- » Largest vessel
- » Can have a WIDE variety of symptoms!
- » Supplies part of the frontal lobe
- » Lateral surface of the temporal & parietal lobes
- » Primary motor & sensory areas of the face, throat, hand & arm
  - Not as much in the legs
- » Supplies some areas of speech

## Complete MCA strokes typically cause:

- Hemiplegia of the contralateral side, affecting the lower part of the face, arm, & hand while largely sparing the leg
- Contralateral (opposite-side) sensory loss in the same areas
- Contralateral homonymous hemianopia***
  - Visual-field deficit affecting the same half of the visual field in both eyes

## Anterior cerebral artery (ACA)

- Not as common
- Branches off the internal carotid artery
- Supplies the anterior-medial portions of the frontal & parietal lobes
  - Controls logical thought, personality & voluntary movement
- Classic symptoms:
  - Contralateral leg motor weakness & sensory loss
  - Evaluate lower-extremity strength & sensation
  - Behavioral abnormalities
  - Incontinence

## Posterior communicating artery (PCA)

- Supplies the inferior & medial temporal & medial occipital lobes
- VISUAL field loss!!!!
- Common - contralateral homonymous hemianopia
- Larger PCA strokes also may cause contralateral hemiparesis & hemi-sensory loss
- Large left PCA strokes may result in aphasia, where-as right PCA strokes may cause neglect

## Basilar artery

- Can affect the cerebellum, brain stem or both
- Symptoms can vary depending where the stroke occurs

## Cerebellar Artery

- Less common (<10%)
- Usually affects one side or section
    - "Cerebellar Syndrome"
- Controls movement & balance
- Each side of cerebellum controls movement for the corresponding side of the body
- Symptoms:
    - Uncoordinated movements of the limbs or trunk
    - Difficulty walking, including problems with balance
    - Assess for limb ataxia
    - Abnormal reflexes
    - Tremors
    - Vertigo —a feeling of spinning or whirling when you are not moving
    - Nausea & vomiting
    - Intense headache
    - Uncontrollable eye movements
    - Swallowing difficulties

## Brain Stem Strokes

- Rare, but can be devastating!!
- Critically ill & often require emergency intubation/ mechanical ventilation
- Symptoms may include:
    - Hemiparesis or tetraplegia
    - Sensory loss affecting either the hemi-body (half of the body) or all four limbs
    - Double vision
    - Dysconjugate gaze
    - Slurred speech
    - Impaired swallow
    - Decreased LOC
    - Abnormal respirations

| Direct Oral Anticoagulation (DOAC) – FYI only | | | | |
|---|---|---|---|---|
| **Drug:** | **Works on:** | **Half-life:** | **FDA approval:** | **Reversal:** |
| Dabigatran (Pradaxa) | DTI, anti-factor IIa | 12 – 17 hours | Non-Valvular afib, VTE Prophylaxis | Praxbind (idarucizumab) |
| Rivaroxaban (Xarelto) | Factor Xa inhibitor | 7 – 11 hours | Non-Valvular afib, VTE prevention | Andexxa (Andexanet alfa) |
| Apixaban (Eliquis) | Factor Xa inhibitor | 12 hours | Venous thromboembolic events | Andexxa (Andexanet alfa) |
| Edoxaban (Lixiana) | Factor Xa inhibitor | 10 – 14 hours | VTE Prophylaxis after ortho surgery, stroke prevention | None available |
| Betrixaban (Bevyxxa) | Factor Xa inhibitor | | VTE, DVT/PE (hospitalized patients) | None available |

# Complications of Stroke:

## Hydrocephalus

» Accumulation of CSF in the ventricles

**Symptoms:**

» Headache

» Decreased LOC, sleepy, confused

» Signs of increased ICP

» Seizures

**Emergent treatment:**

- » Short term: Ventriculostomy
- » Long term: VP Shunt
  - Ventricle to pleural space or ventricle to peritoneal space

**Potential complications of any neuro insult:**

- » Hyponatremia
  - Often caused from SIADH or Cerebral Salt Wasting
  - Na+ < 130 is common
  - Leads to cerebral edema
- » Hypernatremia
- » Diabetes Insipidus
  - Deficiency of ADH
- » Pulmonary complications
  - Aspiration
  - Airway protection
- » Seizures
- » DVT – common!
  - Immobility
  - Heparin prophylaxis OK if stable 3 – 5 days after bleed

# Seizures

- » Abnormal electrical discharges in the brain
- » Duration can range from a few seconds to continuous without intervention
- » > 5 minutes is considered a medical emergency

**Causes:**

- » Genetic
- » Congenital
- » Exposure to drugs
- » Withdrawal from drugs or alcohol
- » Low sodium or glucose
- » Infection
- » Trauma
- » Tumors

## Tonic-clonic (Grand mal) seizures:

### Tonic phase:

- Lose consciousness
- Many times experience a fall
- Rigid extremities
- Bite tongue
- Pupils dilate

### Clonic phase:

- Tachycardia
- Diaphoretic
- Frothing at mouth
- Violent, rhythmic shaking
- Alternating contraction & relaxation

### Postictal phase:

- Altered LOC after seizure
- Lasts between 5 – 30 minutes, sometimes longer
- Drowsiness, confusion, hypertension, headache

## Status Epilepticus

- Seizure lasts more than 30 min
- 20 – 30% mortality
- Safety is a priority!!!
  - Monitor for patent airway
  - Don't ever stick anything into the mouth!!!
- Identify the underlying cause
  - Consider toxicology screen
  - Assess electrolytes & glucose

### Medications - All Seizures

- **Benzodiazepines - #1 priority!**
  - **Lorazepam (Ativan) IV*** (preferred – 1st line)
    - 0.1 mg/kg
    - Repeat in 5 – 10 min
  - Diazepam (Valium)
    - 0.15 mg/kg IV/PR
    - Repeat in 5 minutes
  - Midazolam (Versed)
    - 0.2 mg/kg IV/IM
    - Buccal/intranasal
- Phenytoin (Dilantin)
  - Load 10 - 15 mg/kg or 15 - 20 mg/kg
  - Give slowly! 50 mg/min
  - Peak blood levels in 15 - 20 min
  - Monitor for bradycardia & hypotension
  - Assess levels; 10 – 20 mcg/L therapeutic level
  - Use a filter
  - Monitor IV site for infiltration
- Fosphenytoin
  - 150 mg/min
- Valproic acid

# Guillain-Barré Syndrome

- Autoimmune disorder
- Immune system attacks the peripheral nervous system
- Many times follows when recovering from an illness or <u>virus</u>
- Usually 1 - 3 weeks after
- Temporary damage to the myelin sheath
- Impulses travel slow causing slow movements or ascending paralysis
- Peak incidence age 30 - 40

### Symptoms:

- Paresthesia (numbness & tingling)
- Pins & needles hands, feet & face
- Uncoordinated movements
- Blurred vision
  - Unilateral or bilateral
- Loss of DTRs/areflexia

» Difficulty breathing if diaphram affected

» Muscle weakness usually starts in legs, then arms, face & respiratory

» Ascending paralysis

## Diagnosis:

» Lumbar puncture

» Albuminocytologic dissociation in the CSF

» High protein level, few cells

## Treatment options:

» Plasmapheresis

» IVIG (immunoglobulin)

» It is not understood exactly why either treatment works

## Supportive treatment:

» DVT prophylaxis

» Nutritional support

» Physical Therapy

» Neurogenic bowel & bladder

» Prevent infections!!!

» Psychosocial support

» Airway, monitor for respiratory failure

- ~ 30% require mechanical ventilation

» Recovery weeks to months

# Meningitis

» Inflammation of the meninges

## Symptoms:

» Headache

» Nuchal rigidity

» Fever

» Altered LOC

» Photophobia, phonophobia

» + Brudzinski's sign

- Severe neck stiffness causes a patient's hips & knees to flex when the neck is flexed

» + Kernig's sign

- Severe stiffness of the hamstrings causes an inability to straighten the leg when the hip is flexed to 90 degrees

## Diagnosis:

» Lumbar puncture

» If it's viral meningitis, the results will show:

- + Protein in CSF
- Normal glucose in CSF
- Lymphocytes
- Enteroviruses, herpes simplex virus, varicella zoster virus, HIV

» If it's bacterial meningitis, the results will show:

- +++ Protein in CSF
- Low glucose in CSF
- Neutrophils, WBCs
- Rash may indicate meningococcal infection
- Neisseria meningitis & streptococcus pneumoniae 80% of cases

## Lumbar puncture FYIs:

» Usually L4 – L5 interspace

» Assess "opening pressure", normal: 6 – 18 mm Hg

### CSF sample to assess:

- WBC, RBC, Protein, glucose, gram stain
  - CSF glucose is usually 40% higher than serum
  - Bacterial meningitis—divide CSF glucose by serum glucose
    - Index ≤ 0.4
  - Assess for lactate
    - Increased level = Bacterial
- Supine position post LP

# Hypoxic-Ischemic Brain Injury

- aka "anoxic injury"
- Loss of distinction between gray & white matter in the cerebral hemispheres
  - Happens after cardiac or respiratory arrests & asphyxiation
- Global brain ischemia caused from cessation of cerebral blood flow
- Major injury happens during reperfusion

### Treatment:

- Targeted temperature management to minimize reperfusion injury
- Neuro-protection**

### What happens during arrest & reperfusion?

- Depleted stores of $O_2$ & glucose
- Intracellular calcium influx
- Formation of $O_2$ free radicals
- Release of glutamate
- Intracellular acidosis
- Disruption in blood brain barrier
- Mitochondrial injury
- Apoptosis

### Targeted Temperature Management:

- Only in patients remaining comatose post cardiac arrest
  - Done in the ICU
- Reason: neuro-protection
- 32 – 36° C for 24 hours
- Slow re-warming back to normal temperature
- Avoid fevers post TTM therapy
- Short term memory loss is common
- Monitor electrolytes post TTM

## Traumatic Brain Injuries (TBI)

### Types

- Blunt
- Penetrating
- Blast

### Focal

- Coup-countrecoup
- Contusions
- Lacerations
- Arterial or venous tears

### Causes

- Motor Vehicle Crash
- Assault
- Falls

### Diffuse Brain Injuries "Shearing injury"

- Twist & turn of axons/ shearing injury
- Mild—concussion
  - Usually < 15 min alteration in LOC
  - Stretch injury of the axons
  - Attention span & memory affected (cortical function)
  - Confusion & disorientation after injury
  - Symptoms usually improve after 15 – 30 min
  - Nausea, vomiting, dizziness, headache
  - Can last for a few days

- » Severe—Diffuse Axonal Injury
  - Acceleration/deceleration injury
  - Damage to axons
  - Disconnects the cerebral hemisphere from the reticular activating system (RAS)
  - Coma, often involves the brainstem
  - Increased ICP
  - Cerebral edema
  - Fever
  - Poor prognosis
  - Treatment is supportive

# Skull Fractures

## Signs of a skull fracture:

- » Headache
- » Nausea/vomiting
- » Blurred vision
- » Restlessness, irritability
- » Disequilibrium
- » Nuchal rigidity—stiff neck
- » Pupils sluggish or not reacting to light
- » Confusion
- » Drowsiness

## Key assessment: Is the dura torn?

- » CT Scan (most common) or MRI
  - Yes → surgery to remove bone fragments
- » Monitor for CSF leak
- » High risk of infection

## Types of skull fractures:

### Linear skull fracture

- » Dura usually intact
- » No treatment required

### Depressed skull fracture

» If less than thickness of the skull, no intervention

» If > thickness of skull (~6 mm), will need decompression (OR)

### Basilar skull fracture

» Fracture in the floor of the skull

» Risk of injury to cranial nerves

» Avoid NASOGASTRIC or ORAL TUBES!!

- Avoid oral suctioning

» Battle sign

- Ecchymosis on mastoid bone

» Raccoon eyes

- Ecchymosis around eyes

» Rhinorrhea

- Torn blood vessels in the nose
- CSF can leak; indicates rupture of the meninges
- C/O salty taste from the $Na^+$ in CSF

» Otorrhea

- Test for glucose, + glucose = CSF
- "Halo" sign—place fluid on gauze, if iridescent halo, likely CSF

» Pneumocephalus—air in head

- Also look for other injuries (Subdural hematoma, contusions)
- Treatment HOB flat (if able)
- High concentration oxygen; dissolves the nitrogen in the air

# Acute Epidural Hematoma

» Neuro emergency!!!!—arterial bleed

» Usually temporal or parietal region

» Laceration of meningeal artery &/or vein

» Caused from trauma

### Presentation:

- Loss of consciousness → lucid, if decompensates: coma
- Nausea, vomiting, agitation, confusion
- Severe decompensation – Uncal (lateral) herniation
- Pupils uneven
- Stat Operating Room or Interventional Radiology

## Subdural Hematoma (SDH)

- Bleeding between the dura mater & the arachnoid space
- Elderly are at risk especially if on anticoagulation
- All types of SDH can develop spontaneously r/t anticoagulation therapy

### Acute SDH

- Symptoms hours to days
- Decreased LOC
- Signs of increased ICP
- Ipsilateral occulomotor paralysis
- Contralateral hemiparesis

### Sub-acute SDH

- Hematoma can form 2 days - 2 weeks after initial injury
- Hematoma can cause major brain compression & secondary injury

### Chronic SDH

- Re-bleed weeks following injury
- Elderly
- Headaches
- Confusion

## Epidural & subdural hematoma diagnosis:

- CT Scan—Gold standard
- MRI—If stable
- Angiography—if arterial dissection suspected

### Complications associated with TBI

- Hyponatremia
- Cerebral salt wasting
- SIADH
- Hypernatremia
- Diabetes insipidus
- Pulmonary complications/ aspiration
- Seizures
- Immobility
- DVT

Know how to monitor for each of these!

## Herniation:

### Signs of Supratentorial (Uncal) herniation

- Uncus pressure on the tentorial notch
- Compression of the midbrain
- Change in LOC
- Unilateral pupil dilation
- Lateral displacement

### Infratentorial herniation

- Downward pressure toward brainstem & medulla
- Cushing's response:
  - Bradycardia
  - Systolic hypertension with wide pulse pressure
  - Irregular respirations
- Small pupils
- Ataxic respirations
- Coma

## Posturing:

### Decorticate (Flexion)

- Flexion of the arms, wrist & fingers
- Internal rotation of the lower extremities

### Decerebrate (Extension)

- Arch the back
- Arms extended & pronated
- Primitive response

You can do it!

# Pulmonary Review

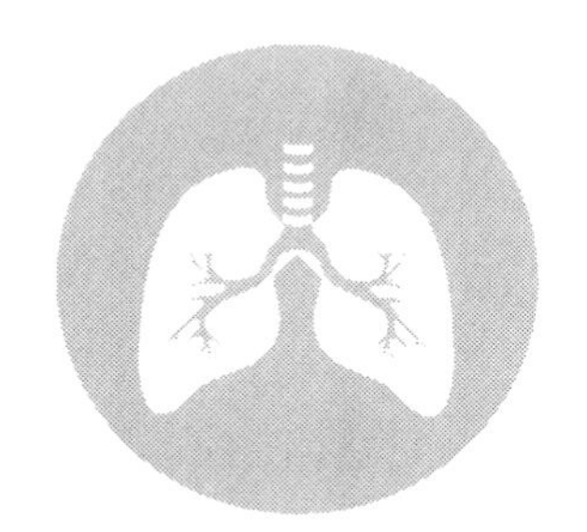

## AACN Test Plan for the Pulmonary portion of the PCCN® Exam

- Acute respiratory distress syndrome (ARDS)
- Asthma (severe)
- COPD exacerbation
- Minimally-invasive thoracic surgery (VATS)
- Obstructive sleep apnea
- Pleural space complications
    - Pneumothorax, hemothorax, pleural effusion, empyema, chylothorax
- Pulmonary embolism
- Pulmonary hypertension
- Respiratory depression
    - Medication induced, decreased LOC induced
- Respiratory failure
    - Acute, chronic, failure to wean
- Respiratory infections
    - Pneumonia
- Thoracic surgery
    - Lobectomy, pneumonectomy

# General Assessment

**Adventitious lung sounds:**

- Crackles (rales)—fluid; heart failure, effusions, pneumonia
- Wheezes—narrowed airways (note if inspiration / expiration)
- Rhonchi (coarse)—Secretions in large airways, pneumonia
- Stridor—obstruction of larynx; harsh high pitched vibrating sound

# Arterial Blood Gases

Know the norms!

Normal blood gas values:

| | |
|---|---|
| **pH:** | 7.35 – 7.45 |
| **$PaO_2$:** | 80 – 100 (on room air) |
| **$PaCO_2$:** | 35 – 45 |
| **$HCO_3$:** | 22 – 26 |
| **Base Deficit:** | -2 to +2 |
| **$SaO_2$:** | 95 – 100% |

Lungs: Fast compensation

Kidneys: Slow compensation

pH < 7.35 leans toward acidosis, > 7.45 leans toward alkalosis

$PaCO_2$ < 35 leans toward alkalosis, > 45 leans toward acidosis

$HCO_3$ < 22 leans toward acidosis, > 26 leans toward alkalosis

Be methodical when interpreting ABGs:

- Look at 3 main values to interpret acid/base balance: pH, $PaCO_2$, $HCO_3$

## Easy method for ABG interpretation:

» Every ABG will have a first name, middle name & last name

Example: pH = 7.31, $PaCO_2$ = 54, $PaO_2$ = 97, $HCO_3$ = 24

1. First name: assess the pH
   - Is it normal or abnormal?
     - 7.31 = abnormal
     - Abnormal = Uncompensated
2. Last name: assess the pH again
   - Is it leaning toward acidosis or alkalosis?
     - 7.31 = Acidosis
3. Middle name: assess the $PaCO_2$ & $HCO_3$
   - Which one is leaning toward acidosis?
     - The $PaCO_2$ is! (Respiratory)
   - If the $PaCO_2$ is the cause the middle name will be respiratory
   - If the $HCO_3$ was the cause, the middle name would be metabolic

» Interpretation: uncompensated respiratory acidosis

## Another tip...

» Look at the pH & $CO_2$

**If the pH & $CO_2$ are both up or both down, it's a metabolic issue!**

- Sa**ME** = **Me**tabolic

Example: pH 7.32 (↓) $CO_2$: 32 (↓) $HCO_3$: 18 $HCO_3$: 18 = metabolic acidosis

**If the pH & $CO_2$ are opposite, it's a respiratory issue!**

- **Re**verse = **Re**spiratory

Example: pH: 7.28 (↓) $CO_2$: 54 (↑) $HCO_3$: 26 = respiratory acidosis

**ROME—Respiratory Opposite, Metabolic Equal**

## Examples:

- pH 7.36 $PaCO_2$ 48 $HCO_3$ 24
  **Compensated Respiratory Acidosis**
- pH 7.26 $PaCO_2$ 35 $HCO_3$ 16
  **Uncompensated Metabolic Acidosis** (pH & $HCO_3$ lean toward acid)
- pH 7.30 $PaCO_2$ 58 $HCO_3$ 30
  **Partially Compensated Respiratory Acidosis** (pH & $PaCO_2$ lean toward acid, $HCO_3$ is leaning in opposite direction; change 1st name to partially compensated)

## Respiratory Acidosis Example

- pH 7.22 $PaCO_2$ 65 $HCO_3$ 24
  **Uncompensated Respiratory Acidosis**

## Respiratory Acidosis Causes:

- Late respiratory failure
- Over-sedation
- Drug overdoses that cause respiratory depression
- COPD
- Brain stem dysfunction
- Acute pulmonary edema
- Extreme V/Q mismatch, Pulmonary embolus, PNA
- Guillain Barré Syndrome
- Excessive $CO_2$ production (Sepsis, TPN, burns)
- Severe obesity
- Think hypoventilation! (retaining $CO_2$)

## Respiratory Alkalosis Example:

- pH 7.52 $PaCO_2$ 26 $HCO_3$ 22
  **Uncompensated Respiratory Alkalosis**

## Respiratory Alkalosis Causes:

- Early respiratory failure
- Anxiety or severe pain
- Increased minute ventilation
- ARDs
- Heart failure
- Fever
- Asthma/emphysema
- Neurologic disorders
- Pulmonary embolus
- Salicylate overdose (adults)
- Decreased cardiac output/shock
- $PaO_2$ < 60 (cause & effect)
- Think hyperventilation! (blowing off $CO_2$)

## Metabolic Acidosis Example:

- pH 7.26 $PaCO_2$ 35 $HCO_3$ 18
  **Uncompensated Metabolic Acidosis**

## Metabolic Acidosis Causes:

- Acute kidney injury
- Drug & alcohol overdoses
- Diabetic ketoacidosis
- Sepsis
- Lactic acidosis
- Toxins
- Aspirin overdose
- Liver failure
- Hyperkalemia, hyperchloremia
- Either the body is producing too much acid, OR
- Kidneys aren't getting rid of it
- Suppresses myocardial contractility
  - ↓ CO, ↓ BP

» Calculate an anion gap!!!

- **Anion gap: normal < 11 – 12**
  - > 12—associated with metabolic acidosis
- Easy acronym for common causes of metabolic acidosis:

**M**: Methanol
**U**: Uremia
**D**: DKA
**P**: Propylene glycol
**I**: Isoniazid
**L**: Lactic Acidosis
**E**: Ethylene glycol
**S**: Salicylates

### Metabolic Alkalosis Example:

- pH 7.49 $PaCO_2$ 36 $HCO_3$ 29
  **Uncompensated Metabolic Alkalosis**

### Metabolic Alkalosis Causes:

- NG tube to suction
- Emesis
- Hypokalemia
- Hypochloremia
- Antacid abuse
- Excessive sodium bicarb infusion
- Inadequate renal perfusion
- Diuretics
- Excessive albuterol use
- Hyperaldosteronism (d/t RAAS activation)
- Too much bicarb in the blood OR,
- Loss of chloride
  - Vomiting – loss of stomach acid

# Hypoxemia

## Three main reasons:

» Hypoventilation

- ↓ minute ventilation
- ↓ Phosphate or magnesium levels
- Obstructive sleep apnea

» Ventilation/perfusion (V/Q) mismatch

- PE, pneumonia, shunt

» Oxygen delivery & consumption imbalance

- ↓ Cardiac output
- Severe anemia

## Intrapulmonary Shunt

» V/Q mismatch

» Excessive blood flow in relation to ventilation

» Ventilation with decreased perfusion

- Increased dead space
- PE is a classic example

## Examples of shunting:

- » Asthma—small airways restricted
- » Pulmonary edema—alveoli filled with fluid
- » Atelectasis—alveolar collapse
- » Pulmonary embolus—non-embolized regions of the lungs (lots of deadspace!)
- » $PaO_2$ decreases as shunt increases

## Oxygen

- » Too much is NOT a good thing!
- » Too little is also NOT a good thing!
- » $O_2$ is a vasoconstrictor in all vascular beds except the lungs (vasodilator)
- » Extensive oxygen can have negative inotropic effects on the heart

## Delivery Methods

- » Nasal cannula 1 - 6 lpm
  - 21% to 46% $FiO_2$
  - High flow cannula
- » Face Mask 5 - 10 lpm
  - 40% to 60% $FiO_2$
- » Partial re-breather mask 5 - 7 lpm
  - 35% to 75% $FiO_2$
- » Non-rebreather mask 5 - 10 lpm
  - 40% to 100% $FiO_2$

# Capnography—$PEtCO_2$

- Normal Capnography is 35 – 45 mm Hg
- Is a measure of ventilation, but also a reflection of perfusion & metabolism
  - If cardiac output drops, capnography values will drop
- Continuous with waveform
- $PEtCO_2$ should be within 5 mm Hg of $PaCO_2$
- Is the gold standard method to verify endotracheal tube placement
  - Lungs vs. gut...still need a chest x-ray to determine how high or low ET tube is
- Standard of care for moderate to deep sedation
  - Hypoventilation = ↑ $EtCO_2$
  - Hyperventilation = ↓ $EtCO_2$
- Used with PCA pumps to identify ineffective ventilation
- Helpful to calculate deadspace & V/Q matching in certain conditions, like:
  - Pulmonary embolus
  - Pneumonia
  - Asthma or COPD exacerbation
- As a measure of perfusion, capnography is helpful with:
  - Resuscitation (CPR quality & ROSC)
  - Low cardiac output states = low $PEtCO_2$
  - Correlation between $PEtCO_2$ & Cardiac Output
  - In cardiac arrest, goal > 10 mm Hg
  - $PEtCO_2$ ↓ in low cardiac output states
  - Mismatched correlation between $PEtCO_2$ & Cardiac Output
    - $PaCO_2$ will be higher

# Acute Respiratory Failure

## Oxygen or ventilation disturbance

Q > V (Perfusion exceeds ventilation)

## Signs:

- Increased work of breathing
- Use of accessory muscles
- Increased minute ventilation
  - Minute ventilation = tidal volume x RR
  - Normal = 5 - 10 L/min
  - Compensating for: increased dead space
- Hallmark sign of late failure:
  - Increased $PaCO_2$/Hypercapnia!!!

## Who is at risk? (Many patients!)

- COPD
- Pneumonia
- Pulmonary edema
- ARDS
- Drug overdoses
- Restrictive lung disease

# Asthma

## Characteristics:

- Airway hyperactivity
- Inflammation
- Bronchial constriction
- Excessive mucus production
- Air trapping with hyperinflation of the lungs
- Lots of resistance!
- Air trapping leads to ↑AUTO-PEEP
  - Increased pressure in distal airways

## Treatment:

- 1st Line Therapy: BRONCHODILATORS!!!!
- aka - $Beta_2$ agonist
- Albuterol—onset < 5 min
  - Effects last 2 - 5 hours
  - Repetitive or continuous albuterol nebs:
    - 2.5 mg per treatment
    - Continuous: 5 - 15 mg/hr

## Side effects of Albuterol:

- Tachycardia
- Tremors (stimulates $Beta_2$ receptors)
- Hyperglycemia
- Hypokalemia
- Hypomagnesemia
- Hypophosphatemia

# Other asthma treatments:

## Anticholinergic Agents

- Ipratropium bromide (Atrovent)
- Derivative of atropine
- Used only in combination with $Beta_2$ agonist (like albuterol)
- Conflicting evidence
- Used in severe exacerbation
- 0.5 mg neb every 20 min x 3, then every 2 – 4 hours
- MDI 4 – 8 puffs

## Corticosteroids

- Reduces secondary airway inflammation & edema
- Prevents relapse
- Methylprednisolone or prednisone for ≤ 7 days
- Neither PO or IV is superior, benefit not seen until 12 hours after therapy started
- No need to taper
- Monitor for myopathies

### Other thoughts on asthma treatment:

- No $O_2$ unless ↓ $O_2$ sats
- No CXR unless suspect PNA
- No ABG unless non-responsive to therapy
- No antibiotics unless there is an infection!
- Hydration is key!
- Hypercapnia is an ominous sign
- Can consider Magnesium Sulfate 1 - 2 grams over 2 hours
    - Bronchodilation effects
- Heliox (helium & oxygen combination)
    - Decreases airway resistence & turbulance
    - Decreases work of breathing
    - 70:30 or 60:40
        - Helium:oxygen

## Chronic Obstructive Pulmonary Disease (COPD)

- Umbrella term for emphysema & chronic bronchitis
- Constant airflow obstruction
- Cough, +/- Sputum
- Worsens over time
- Shortness of breath
- Diagnosis: Pulmonary Function Test
    - $FEV_1/FVC$
    - Normal = 80%

### Other characteristics of COPD—Emphysema

- Air-trapping with chronic hyperinflation of lungs
- Prolonged exhalation
- Barrel chest
- Clubbed fingers
- Enlarged right heart
- Elevated right sided venous pressures (CVP)
- Develop intrinsic PEEP (high pressure) from chronic air trapping

## COPD Exacerbation Treatment:

- Most common reason for exacerbation is upper respiratory infections
- Bronchodilators—some thought there may be limited benefit
- Short course of corticosteroids — ≤ 7 days
  - Methylprednisolone or prednisone
  - No advantage of IV over PO
  - Inhaled steroids longterm & bronchodilators
- Antibiotics are debated as many infections are viral
  - Strep pneumonia
  - H. flu
  - Problem: antibiotic resistance
- Oxygen therapy general guideline:
  - Keep $O_2$ sats low 90% range, avoid high concentration of $O_2$
  - If $O_2$ needed, monitor for signs of hypercapnia & decreased LOC
- Non-invasive ventilation
  - CPAP for hypoxic failure
  - Bi-Pap for hypercapnic failure
- Intubate if:
  - Respiratory distress with hemodynamic compromise
  - Mental status change, somnolence
  - Worsening acidosis
  - Monitor for intrinsic PEEP (Auto-PEEP)
    - Increased pressure in distal airways

## COPD vs. Asthma

- COPD
  - Onset in mid-life
  - Symptoms slowly progressive
  - Long smoking history
- Asthma
  - Onset early in life (often childhood)
  - Symptoms vary from day to day
  - Symptoms worse at night/ early morning
  - Allergy, rhinitis, &/or eczema also present
  - Family history of asthma

## Non-Invasive Positive Pressure Ventilation (NPPV)

### CPAP/BiPAP

- Continuous positive pressure
- Stabilizes airways during exhalation
- Improves ventilation (BiPap)
- Keeps alveoli open
- Used to treat:
  - COPD exacerbation
  - CHF, pulmonary edema
  - Obstructive sleep apnea
  - Obesity hypoventilation syndrome
- Monitor for facial skin breakdown

### CPAP

- Simple mask & $O_2$
- Set at 5 – 10 cm $H_2O$
- Increases functional residual capacity
  - Volume in the lungs at end—exhalation
- Does not augment tidal volume

### Bi-PAP

- Bi-level positive airway pressure
- CPAP that alternates between 2 pressure levels
- Higher mean airway pressures, more alveolar recruitment
- Provides larger tidal volumes
- Set IPAP & EPAP
- Typical starting point:
  - IPAP 10 cm $H_2O$, EPAP 5 cm $H_2O$
  - Inspiratory time 0.8 - 2 seconds

# Pulmonary Embolus

- 70% have a DVT
  - Usually from deep venous system of lower extremities
- Alveoli are ventilated, but there is a lack of perfusion
  - V/Q mismatch
- Most emboli are multiple
- Lower lobes of lung are more commonly involved with emboli vs. upper lobes
- Excessive dead space
  - Air that doesn't take part in gas exchange

## Risk factors:

- **Immobility**
- Surgery
- Trauma
- Clotting disorders
- Hemolytic anemia

## Signs:

- Tachycardia
- Tachypnea
- Dyspnea
- Chest pain
- Crackles
- Diaphoresis
- Hemoptysis
- Sudden right heart failure
- Increased pulmonary artery pressures
- PEA Arrest
  - Dilated RV compresses LV

## Diagnosis

- Spiral (helical) CT scan—detector rotated around the patient; 2-D view
  - 30 seconds or less to perform scan
  - Hold breath at intervals during scan
  - Contrast infused to view pulmonary vasculature
  - 93% sensitivity / 97% specificity if clot is in one of the main arteries

## Other diagnostics:

- » Pulmonary angiogram
  - Most accurate
  - Performed in < 20% of patients with PE because it takes too long
- » Ultrasound—DVT extremities
- » V/Q Scan—only diagnoses 25 – 30% of cases
  - Underlying lung disease—abnormal scan
- » 12 Lead ECG findings:
  - Not specific to PE
  - Right axis deviation
  - Transient right BBB
  - ST depression, T wave depression in $V_1 - V_4$
  - Tall peaked T waves in II, III, aVF
- » ABG—low $PaO_2$

## Treatment:

### If hemodynamically stable:

- » Unfractionated Heparin (UFH)
  - Weight-based dosing
  - Prevent progression
  - Bolus, then continuous infusion
  - Goal: aPTT 50 – 80 seconds (Some hospitals target 60 - 100)
- » Warfarin
  - Used with UFH
  - Usually start on 1st day of Heparin therapy
  - Goal: INR 2 – 3, then d/c Heparin
  - Continue for a minimum of 6 weeks or more

## Can also use:

- » Low Molecular Weight Heparin (LMWH)
- » Fondaparinux
- » Enoxaparin 1 mg/kg Q 12 hours
  - Cleared by the kidneys (renal adjustment)
  - Simplified dosing
  - No need to monitor coags
  - Treat outpatient
- » EKOS Catheter w/rtPA

**If the patient has hemodynamic instability or cardiac arrest:**

- Fibrinolytic therapy
  - Alteplase (rtPA)
  - Reteplase
  - 12% chance of major hemorrhage
  - 1% ICH
  - Have to weigh benefit > risk

### IVC Filters

**Used for DVT if:**

- Contraindication to anticoagulation
- Pulmonary embolus while on anticoagulation
- Thrombus in right heart or free floating
- No DVT, but ↑ risk of hemorrhage

## Pulmonary Arterial Hypertension (PAH)

- High pressure in the pulmonary vasculature
- Leads to right sided heart failure

**Causes:**

- Idiopathic
- Medications
- Systemic hypertension
- Obstructive sleep apnea (OSA)
- Sclerotic diseases
- Lung diseases

**Common treatments for symptomatic PAH (oral):**

- Sildenafil (Viagra)
- Bosentan (Tracleer)
  - Both are pulmonary vasodilators

### Rapid progression treatment:

- Epoprostenol (Flolan)—Continuous IV (short half-life)
  - Always have an extra bag on standby
- Treprostinil (Remodulin)
- Goal with all meds is pulmonary vasodilation
- Watch for hypotension

# Lung Cancer

- Patients often present with c/o cough, shortness of breath, hemoptysis, fatigue, weight loss
- Diagnosed usually by chest radiograph → CT scan → biopsy

### Treatment - 3 common types of surgery:

- Wedge resection
  - Small wedge of lung tissue removed
- Lobectomy
  - A lobe of the lung is removed
- Pneumonectomy
  - Entire lung removed from one side
  - May also remove lymph nodes

### Post-Operative Treatment Strategies:

#### Fluids

- DO NOT FLUID OVERLOAD!!!!
  - In the first 24 hours, usually give < 20 ml/kg TOTAL fluid
- Monitor for pulmonary edema:
  - More common with right pneumonectomy
- Right pneumonectomy patients have challenges
  - The right carries > 50% of lung volume & vasculature
- Lower hemoglobin may be OK in this population
  - Usually don't transfuse unless the Hgb < 7g/dL & they are symptomatic

## Pain

- Big issue!!!!
- Pain can last for months after surgery
- After OR, use a multi-modal approach
    - Epidural or nerve blocks
    - NSAIDs, acetaminophen, ketamine, Gabapentin

## Chest tubes:

- Will have a prolonged air leak
    - Remain in place until the air leak has resolved
    - Often placed to water seal
    - For pneumonectomy: NEVER place CT to suction!
- May see mediastinal shift
- If there is sudden bleeding, contact the provider STAT!
    - Will need to return to surgery
    - Assess for coagulopathy

## Positioning:

- Out of bed as much as possible
- DVT prophylaxis
- Position operative lung DOWN, good lung UP!!!
    - Promotes fluid filling of the removed lung

## Cardiovascular events:

- Monitor for cardiac ischemia
- Atrial fibrillation in up to 30% of patients!
    - Don't usually use Amiodarone for pneumonectomy due to pulmonary toxicity side effects
    - Use beta blockers, Diltiazem
    - If lobectomy can use BB, Dilt or Amio

## Other post-operative concerns:

- Atelectasis!!!
    - Cough, deep breath, incentive spirometry
    - Chest PT if needed
    - Early mobility is a MUST!

# Pulmonary Contusion

## Mechanism of Injury

- Damage to the parenchyma of the lung
- Localized edema
- Hemorrhage, rupture capillaries

## Symptoms:

- Not always immediate—24 to 72 hours, once swelling starts!
- Tachypnea
- Tachycardia
- Hypoxemia
- Hemoptysis—pink, frothy
- Crackles
- External signs of ecchymosis, rib fractures

## Diagnosis:

- CT scan—most sensitive
- Differentiate between atelectasis & aspiration
- ↓ P/F ratio
    - $PaO_2 \div FiO_2$
    - Normal = > 300
- ↓ $PaCO_2$ (d/t ↑ RR)
    - Early failure—blow off $CO_2$

## Treatment:

- Supportive with severe contusions, treat like ARDS if hypoxic
- Do not fluid overload!!!

# Rib fractures

- 4 - 8 most common
- 9 - 12 concern with rupture of spleen, liver or diaphragmatic tear
- Diagnosed by chest x-ray
- Pain control—consider epidural catheter
- **Prevent Pneumonia
  - Encourage incentive spirometer

## Hemothorax

- Blood in the pleural space
  - Lung tissue is compressed, collapses alveoli
  - Often accompanied by a pneumothorax

### Causes:

- Trauma, thoracic surgery, thoracic aneurysm
- > 400 mls—symptomatic
- Hypovolemia & shock
- Respiratory acidosis, dropping hemoglobin
- Absent breath sounds on affected side
- CT scan to diagnose
- Place chest tube
- Thoracotomy if unable to control bleeding

## Pneumothorax

- Air in the pleural space

### Causes:

- Trauma
- Too much PEEP
- Ruptured bleb
- Lung disease (COPD, cystic fibrosis, pneumonia)

## 3 types:

- Closed
  - Air enters through airways & cannot escape
  - ↑ Intrathoracic chest pressure
  - ↑ Pressure on lungs & heart → leads to tension pneumothorax
- Tension (the really bad one!)
  - Life threatening
  - Air accumulates in pleural space & cannot escape
  - Pressure collapses the lung
  - Decreased capacity, decreased compliance
  - Can lead to PEA Arrest
- Open
  - Penetrating injury
  - Air enters & exits
  - Less dangerous

## Signs & Symptoms:

- Depends on size
- Dyspnea
- Restlessness
- Anxiety
- Chest pain
- SOB
- Cyanosis
- Decreased or absent breath sounds on affected side
- Tracheal shift toward unaffected side

## Treatment:

- Diagnosed by chest x-ray
- ABG—low $PaO_2$
- If it is small, treatment may not be necessary
  - Air will be reabsorbed
- If larger pneumo, chest tube
- Emergent needle decompression:
  - 14 – 16 gauge needle
  - 2nd ICS, midclavicular line, right above 3rd rib
  - Listen for air escaping

### Chest Tubes:

- Use suction to re-expand the lung
- 10 – 20 cm $H_2O$ suction (or up to 40 cm $H_2O$ with dry suction)
- Follow CXR
- Do NOT milk or strip chest tubes...it can create up to -400 cm $H_2O$ pressure!!!
- Tidaling is normal
  - Fluctuation with breathing in the water seal/air leak chamber
- Spontaneously breathing patient:
  - Water level rises during inspiration, falls during exhalation
  - Opposite for mechanically ventilated patient
  - If tidaling is not present: assess for obstructing in the tubing (clot or kink)

### Signs of a pneumothorax:

- Bubbling in the water seal/ air leak chamber
- Shortness of breath
- First check connections (assessing for a system air leak) – if that doesn't resolve bubbling, it may be a patient air leak
- Chest radiograph will verify if there is a pneumothorax

# Advanced airways

### Endotracheal Tubes

- Oral is preferred placement
  - Can insert nasal
- Smaller number = smaller tube
- Most adult sizes 7.0, 7.5 or 8.0
- Placement confirmed via waveform Capnography**
  - Auscultating the chest is not overly helpful
  - Chest x-ray done to verify placement
  - ET tube should sit 3 – 4 cm above carina (± 2 cm)
- Ideal cuff pressure 20 – 30 cm $H_2O$

### Tracheostomy Tubes

- Used if long term support anticipated
- Emergency—obstruction
- Always have an extra trach at the patient's bedside
- Keep clean—avoid hydrogen peroxide, use saline to clean
- Can deflate the cuff so the patient can talk
    - Use a one-way valve

## Mechanical ventilation

### Basic settings (for emergent intubation):

- Mode of ventilation
    - Ventilator brand dependent, but usually pressure or volume or a combo of both
- Rate (breaths per minute)
    - If the $PaCO_2$ is elevated, can ↑ the rate to blow it off
- Tidal volume
    - Volume of air in/out of lungs
    - Generally 8 mL/kg PBW
    - Based on predicted body weight—if you gain weight your lung size doesn't change!
- PEEP
    - Usually start with 5
- $FiO_2$
    - Less is more!

### Modes of ventilation basics:

- Volume mode:
    - The ventilator delivers a pre-set volume of air with every breath
    - This is the most commonly used mode
- Pressure mode:
    - The ventilator will deliver a breath until a pre-set pressure is reached

### Basic Ventilator Alarms:

- Low pressure alarm: usually a leak or disconnect in the circuit
  - Start with the patient & check all connections
- High pressure alarm: high pressure in the circuit
  - Secretions, water or kinks in the tubing can cause high pressure
- Low Minute Ventilation (Ve): The amount of air inhaled per minute drops below a set value
  - It will act similar to a low-pressure alarm & usually indicates a leak or disconnect in the system

# Acute Respiratory Distress Syndrome (ARDS)

- Inflammatory response in the lungs
- It is not a primary disease, but a result of:
  - Sepsis
  - Trauma
  - Multiple blood transfusions (TRALI, CRALI)
  - Pancreatitis
  - Cardiopulmonary bypass
  - Pulmonary contusion
  - Pneumonia/aspiration

### What is happening in ARDS?

- INFLAMMATORY RESPONSE!
- Alveoli are infiltrated with leukocytes
- Fibrin deposits in lungs
- Widespread endothelial & alveolar damage
- Leaky capillaries
- Lungs get stiff
- Decreased compliance
- Non-cardiogenic pulmonary edema

## Signs:

- » Tachypnea
- » Progressive refractory hypoxemia
- » Worsening P/F ratio
    - $PaO_2 \div FiO_2$
    - Normal is > 300
- » CXR—Bilateral pulmonary infiltrates
- » Usually require mechanical ventilation within 48 hours
- » What therapy will improve the $PaO_2$?
    - Answer: PEEP!

## Diagnosis:

- » Timing: Within 1 week of a known clinical insult
- » Pulmonary infiltrates on CXR
    - Bilateral opacities
- » P/F ratio: $PaO_2 \div FiO_2$

Berlin Criteria—2012

- » P/F ratio:
    - < 300—Mild ARDS
    - < 200—Moderate ARDS
    - < 100—Severe ARDS
- » Predisposing conditions
- » Absence of left heart failure or left atrial hypertension
- » Non-cardiogenic pulmonary edema
- » Mimics pneumonia & cardiogenic pulmonary edema
- » Broncho-alveolar Lavage (BAL) or Bronchoscopy
    - Sample examined for neutrophils & protein
    - Neutrophils: Up to 80% in ARDS
        - ▹ Normal: 5%
    - Higher protein level in aspirate, sign of inflammation

## ARDS Treatment:

- Rest the lungs
- Mechanical ventilation with "Lung Protective Ventilation" or "LPV"
  - Can try BiPap, but mechanical ventilation is inevitable if they decompensate
- Low tidal volumes
  - Start at 6 ml/kg PBW
  - Lowest 4 mL/kg PBW
- Larger tidal volumes over distend & rupture distal air space (volutrauma)
- Limit pressure related injury (barotrauma)
- Use predicted body weight when establishing tidal volume settings
- Use of PEEP
  - Think of PEEP as a stent to keep alveoli open
- When increasing PEEP, monitor for signs of decreased cardiac output!!!
  - May see hypotension
- They need to be in the ICU!

## Other therapies:

- Conservative fluid management
  - Do NOT fluid overload patients!
  - Diuretics
  - Able to liberate the patient from the ventilator quicker!
- Optimize $O_2$ delivery
  - Cardiac Output: Dobutamine if cardiac dysfunction
  - $PaO_2$: PEEP
  - Low hemoglobin: Transfuse only if necessary!
- Steroids
  - No benefit from early steroids
  - Some benefit days 7 – 14
  - Methylprednisolone 2 – 3 mg/kg/day
  - Inhibits fibrinolysis
- Prone positioning—FYI (done in ICU)
  - New evidence of benefit
  - Must be done early, not used as a last ditch treatment
  - Should remain prone > 16 hours per day

# Renal & Electrolytes Review

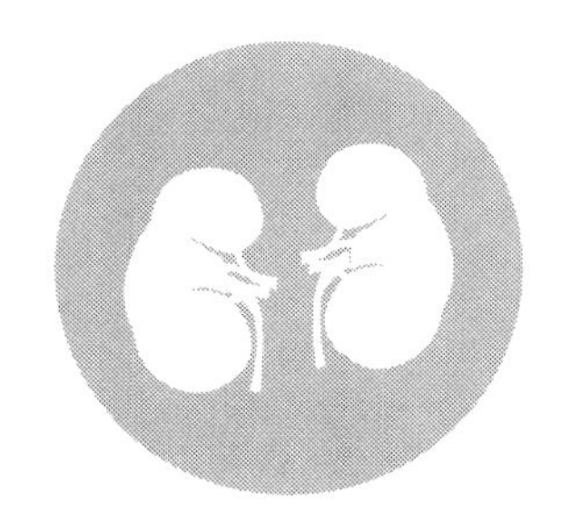

**AACN Test Plan for the Renal & Electrolytes portion of the PCCN® Exam:**

- Acute kidney injury (AKI)
- Chronic kidney disease (CKD)
- End stage renal disease (ESRD)
- Electrolyte imbalances

# Overview of the renal system

- Approximately 20% of cardiac output goes to the kidneys
- Renal arteries branch directly off aorta

## Main function of the kidneys

- Cleanse & detoxify blood
- Filtration
- Reabsorption of water, electrolytes, amino acids
- Secretion of water & wastes
- Acid/base balance
- Blood pressure regulation
- Erythropoietin production

### The nephron is made of the:

- **Glomerulus**
  - Network of capillaries
  - Filters blood
- **Proximal Convoluted Tubule**
  - Reabsorbs $H_2O$, sodium, amino acids & glucose
- **Loop of Henle**
  - Reabsorbs $Na^+$, water & concentrates urine
  - This is where loop diuretics work (i.e. Lasix)
- **Distal Convoluted Tubule**
  - Regulates pH, $K^+$, $Na^+$ & $Ca^{++}$
- **Collecting Duct**
  - Collects urine from the nephrons

### Fluid balance is regulated by:

- Thirst
- Anti-diuretic hormone (ADH)
- Aldosterone
  - Causes retention of $Na^+$ & $H_2O$
  - Elevated $K^+$ triggers release of aldosterone
- Atria-natriuretic peptide (ANP)
  - Overstretch of the atria triggers the kidneys to excrete water
- Renin Angiotensin Aldosterone System (RAAS)
  - When activated, triggers the kidneys to conserve sodium & water

## Urine

- **Normal urine output**
  - 1 – 1.5 L/day or 0.5 mL/kg/hour
- **Anuria**
  - < 100 mL/day
- **Oliguria**
  - < 400 mL/day
- **Polyuria**
  - > 2500 mL/day

## Acute Kidney Injury (AKI)

- a.k.a. Acute renal failure (ARF)
- Abrupt decline in glomerular filtration rate (GFR)
- Results in retention of metabolic waste
  - Protein catabolism (azotemia)
- Electrolyte & acid-base imbalance
  - Retention of potassium, magnesium & phosphate
- Fluid overload
- Acid/base imbalance
  - Metabolic acidosis

### Causes of acute kidney injury:

- Low perfusion, medications, parenchymal disease
- Reversible if prompt treatment is received

### Risk factors for developing AKI

- Elderly
- Heart failure
- Baseline renal insufficiency
- Elevated body mass index (BMI > 32)
- COPD
- Liver disease
- Sepsis
- Medications
- GI Bleeding
- Burns & trauma
- Multi-System Organ Failure
- Hypotension/decreased C.O.
- Rhabdomyolysis
- IV contrast dye
- Hypovolemia for whatever reason

## Common labs in AKI:

- Azotemia—elevated BUN
- Elevated creatinine
  - Up to 12 hour lag time in elevation, not an early indicator!
- BUN/Creatinine ratio, normal ratio is 10:1 to 15:1
- Glomerular Filtration Rate
  - Estimated by creatinine clearance
- Urinalysis:
  - Casts - presence is a sign of tubular cell death
  - Electrolytes (specifically $Na^+$)
  - Albumin
  - Glucose
  - Protein

## Glomerular Filtration Rate (GFR)

- Estimated by assessing creatinine clearance
- The measurement of how much filtrate is made by the kidney (ml/min)
- Normal creatinine clearance is about 80 – 120 ml/min
- It is used to evaluate the kidneys' ability to remove waste products from the body
- Males have a creatinine clearance slightly higher than females
- Isolated plasma creatinine is not a sensitive marker for GFR in early stages of kidney injury

**Equations used to estimate GFR (this is FYI only!):**

- Cockcroft-Gault

$$GFR = (140 - age) \times (weight) / (sCr \times 72)\ (\times 0.85 \text{ for } ♀)$$

OR

- MDRD—Modification of Diet in Renal Disease

$$GFR = 186 \times (\text{serum creatinine in mg/dL})^{-1.154} \times (\text{Age in years})\ -0.203\ (\times 0.742 \text{ if female})\ (\times 1.210 \text{ if African-American})$$

# Acute Kidney Injury (AKI)

### Three Categories of AKI:

## Postrenal AKI

- » Think obstruction!
- » Injury caused by disruption of urine flow
- » Causes: urethral obstruction, prostate disease, infection, neurogenic bladder (i.e. spinal cord injury), blood clots, stones
- » Oliguria
- » BUN & creatinine elevated
- » Normal BUN/Creatinine ratio 10 - 15:1, but both elevated
- » ↑ urine specific gravity, ↑ urine osmo

### Treatment:

- » Relieve obstruction
- » Will likely need bladder catheter

## Prerenal AKI

- » Results from hypoperfusion
- » Kidney structure & function is preserved
- » Causes: Sepsis, heart failure, trauma, severe hypovolemia
- » BUN/Creatinine ratio > 20:1
  - BUN elevates, creatinine may start to elevate
- » Oliguria
- » Urine $Na^+$ < 20 mEq/L
  - Kidneys hold on to $Na^+$ & $H_2O$
- » Urine osmo & urine specific gravity ↑ due to concentration
- » HIGH RISK for progressing to ATN!

### Treatment:

- » Treat cause, improve perfusion

# Acute Tubular Necrosis (ATN)

- May also be referred to "intrarenal" kidney injury
- Injury occurs at the nephron; there is structural damage!
- Causes: Hypotension, glomerulonephritis, diabetes, rhabdomyolysis, nephrotoxic medications, shock states
- BUN > 25 mg/dL, creatinine > 1.2 mg/dL
- BUN/Creatinine ratio 10:1 - 15:1, both BUN & creatinine are elevated
- Often requires renal replacement therapy (RRT)/dialysis

## Treatment:

- Depends on cause, assess if dialysis is indicated
- Prevent & treat acidosis, electrolyte imbalance & uremia
- Stop nephrotoxic medications
- Ensure adequate cardiac output
- Avoid NSAIDs!

# Two types of Acute Tubular Necrosis (ATN):

## Ischemic ATN

- Irregular damage along tubular membranes
- Tubular cell damage & cast formation
- Poor perfusion to kidneys
- Recovery long

## Toxic ATN

- Caused by drugs or bacteria
- Aminoglycosides & antivirals are common offenders
- Uniform, wide spread damage to the renal tubules
- Recovery more rapid (< 8 days)
- ***Reversible if offending cause is stopped!

## Three distinct phases of ATN:

### Oliguric Phase

- Insult to injury within 48 hours
- Inability to excrete fluids & metabolic wastes
- Significant ↑ in BUN & creatinine
- Fluid overload
- Metabolic acidosis
- Electrolyte imbalance (especially $K^+$)
- Urine $Na^+$ < 10 mEq/L
  - Elevated urine specific gravity
- Often requires dialysis

### Diuretic Phase

- Lasts 7 – 14 days
- Gradual improvement in renal function
- ↑ in GFR & often develop polyuria
- Urine output 2 – 5 L/day
- Hemodialysis may cover polyuria
- Kidneys can often clear volume, but not solute or waste
- Waste electrolyte—monitor $K^+$ & $Na^+$ closely!
- ↓ urine specific gravity, ↓ urine osmo
- Monitor for fluid deficit
  - Can lead to secondary injury

### Recovery Phase

- Can progress to CKD
- GFR returns to < 80% of normal within 1 – 2 years

**With all kidney injury, ensure patients:**

1. Have adequate **HYDRATION**
2. Have adequate **PERFUSION**
3. Stop any **NEPHROTOXIC** Meds!

## Summary of each type of failure:

| | Prerenal | (ATN) Intrarenal | Postrenal |
|---|---|---|---|
| Urine Volume | Oliguria | Oliguria in Oliguric phase, polyuria in diuretic phase | Oliguric to anuria |
| Specific Gravity (normal 1.01 – 1.02) | >1.02 | ↑in oliguric phase, ↓in diuretic phase | Normal to elevated |
| Urinary Sodium (normal 40 – 100) | < 20 mEq/L | < 10 mEq/L in oliguric phase, > 20 - 40 mEq/L in diuretic phase | > 40 mEq/L |
| Urinary Sediment | Normal<br>No protein | Erythrocyte and/or tubular casts, hematuria Proteinuria | Possible bacteria |
| BUN to Creatinine ratio (normal 10:1) | > 20:1 | 10:1 – 15:1<br>(both elevated) | 10:1 – 15:1<br>(both elevated) |
| Urine Osmolality (normal 500 - 850) | Elevated - > 500 | Elevated if oliguric;<br>Lower if diuretic phase - < 350 | < 350 |

## List of most nephrotoxic medications:

- Aminoglycoside antibiotics (Gentamycin)
- Amphotericin B
- Cisplatin
- IV contrast dye
- Immunoglobulins
- NSAIDs
- ACE Inhibitors
- ARBs
- Acyclovir
- Triamterene
- Sulphonamides
- Methotrexate
- Beta lactam antibiotics
- Vancomycin
- Rifampicin
- Ciprofloxacin

### Uremic Syndrome symptoms (when the BUN is elevated)

- Neurologic: Lethargy, fatigue, seizures, coma
- Cardiovascular: ECG changes (d/t hyperkalemia), signs of fluid overload; tachycardia, S3 heart sound, hypo/hypertension
- Hematologic: Anemia
- Pulmonary: Crackles, pulmonary edema, SOB, effusions, pleuritis from uremia
- Gastrointestinal: Decreased appetite, nausea & vomiting, ascites & fluid overload

### General Treatment Goals for AKI

- Hemodynamic stability
- Improve renal perfusion
- Correct chemistry abnormalities (electrolytes, BUN, creatinine)
- Monitor electrolytes for imbalances
    - During & after therapy
- Adequate hydration
    - Careful use of diuretics
    - Accurate, meticulous daily weights
- Aggressive dialysis
- Monitor drug levels for toxicity
- Monitor coags
- Alter medication schedules around dialysis if needed
- Modify medication dosing—identify meds cleared through kidneys
- Minimize exposure to nephrotoxic medications
- Prevent infection
- Maintain nutritional state

# Contrast induced nephropathy (CIN)

- Highest risk patients:
    - Diabetics, HTN, heart failure
    - Pre-existing renal insufficiency
    - Dehydrated
    - Concurrent use of nephrotoxic medications (i.e. NSAIDs, some antibiotics)
    - High volume of IV contrast
        - 10% of all patients who receive IV contrast dye develop CIN—yikes!

- ***HYDRATION!!! is the key to prevention
  - A little rhyme to remember: The **solution** to **pollution** (contrast dye) is **dilution**!!!!
  - Hydrate to protect the kidneys!!!
- Sodium bicarbonate infusion—1 hour before & 6 hours after exposure to contrast dye
  - Not much evidence to support this is actually helpful
- N-Acetylcysteine (Mucomyst) for prevention (stinky!)
  - 600 mg PO day before & day of contrast exposure (total of 4 doses)
  - Thought to prevent toxicity to renal tubules
  - Not much evidence to support this

# Chronic Kidney Disease (CKD)

- Slow, progressive deterioration of renal function
- Persistent & progressive reduction in GFR (< 60 ml/min/1.73 $m^2$) &/or albuminuria
- Diminished renal reserve puts patients at higher risk for development

## Lab Findings:

- Anemia
- ↑ BUN, creatinine, phosphate, $K^+$, $Mg^{++}$
- ↓ $Ca^{++}$, bicarb, protein

## Risk Factors for the development of Chronic Kidney Disease (CKD)

- Diabetes*
- Hypertension*
- Autoimmune diseases
- Systemic infection
- Urinary stones or strictures
- Prolonged exposure to nephrotoxic drugs
- Elderly

» Race or ethnic background

» Exposure to chemicals or environmental toxins

» Family history

* Together responsible for 70% of CKD cases

### Stages of Chronic Kidney Disease—mostly FYI

» **Stage 1:** Damage w/ increased GFR
- (> 90 ml/min/1.73 $m^2$)

» **Stage 2:** Mild reduction GFR
- (60 – 89 ml/min/1.73 $m^2$)

» **Stage 3:** Moderate reduction in GFR
- (30 – 59 ml/min/1.73 $m^2$)

» **Stage 4:** Severe reduction in GFR
- (15 – 29 ml/min/1.73 $m^2$)

» **Stage 5:** Kidney Failure
- (< 15 ml/min/1.73 $m^2$)

# Renal Replacement Therapy (RRT)

## Indications for Dialysis

» Easy acronym to remember reasons:

**A**: Acid/base imbalance

**E**: Electrolyte imbalance (hyperkalemia, hypermagnesemia, hyperphosphatemia)

**I**: Intoxications (ODs/toxins)

**O**: Overload (fluid)

**U**: Uremic symptoms

### Laboratory findings in ATN in need of RRT:

- BUN > 35
- Creatinine > 4 or, creatinine climbing ≥ 1 point/day
- Uncompensated metabolic acidosis
- Anemia
- Electrolyte imbalances
  - Increased potassium (> 6.5), magnesium, phosphate
  - Decreased calcium, bicarb
  - Abnormal urine electrolytes

# Dialysis

### Emergent dialysis options:

- Hemodialysis
- Continuous renal replacement therapy (CRRT)—done in ICU
- Peritoneal

#### Principles of Dialysis

- Two compartments (blood & filtrate) separated by a semi-permeable membrane
- Pressure gradients are created
- Water, toxins, electrolytes & drugs can cross the membrane
- Goal is to reach equilibrium on each side of the membrane

#### Hemodialysis

- Intermittent
- Slow Low Efficiency Dialysis (SLED)
  - HD at lower flow rate; usually over 12 hours
- Artificial kidney (hemofilter) with a synthetic membrane
- Dialysate is bicarbonate & sodium based with electrolytes
- Short term access
  - Double lumen catheter
- Long term access
  - AV fistula

## Hemodialysis Complications

- Hypotension
- Dysrhythmias (d/t electrolyte shifts)
- Angina
- Fever from pyrogenic reaction
- Coagulopathy, thrombocytopenia
- Disequilibrium syndrome
  - Post-treatment cerebral edema
- Air embolism (rare)

## A quick acronym to remember medications removed by Dialysis:

- **B** - Barbiturates
- **L** - Lithium
- **I** - Isoniazid
- **S** - Salicylates
- **T** -Theophylline/Caffeine
  - Both are methylxanthines
- **M** - Methanol
- **E** - Ethylene glycol
- **D** – Depakote

Hold BP meds until after dialysis!

## Air Embolism

**Venous signs:**

- Shortness of breath
- Chest pain
- Acute right heart failure
  - If obstructs blood flow from right heart to the lungs
- Looks like a pulmonary embolism!

## Treatment:

- Lay on left side, trendelenburg position
- Hyperoxygenate with 100% $FiO_2$
  - Accelerates the removal of nitrogen in the air embolism
- Hyperbaric oxygen therapy

### Arterial signs:

- Change in LOC (looks like a stroke!)
- Decreased arterial flow & perfusion (looks like an occluded artery)
    - It only takes 2 ml of air to be fatal in an artery
    - Only 0.5 ml air to be fatal in a coronary artery
- Oxygenate with high concentration oxygen to dissolve the nitrogen in the air

## Peritoneal Dialysis (PD)

- Primarily used for long term kidney disease, but can be used in emergencies
- Soft catheter inserted percutaneously into abdominal cavity
- Abdominal mesenteric capillary bed is utilized as the semi-permeable membrane
- Glucose-based dialysate is used
    - 1.5%, 2.5%, 4.25% glucose solutions are often used
    - 4.25% solution is going to pull more fluid off than 1.5%
    - Higher glucose concentration = ↑ fluid removal (via diffusion gradient)
- Usually 2 Liter exchanges done every 3 - 4 hours
- Advantages: patient can do at home, cost effective, no need for anticoagulation or vascular access

### Complications of Peritoneal Dialysis (PD):

- Peritonitis
    - Increased WBCs, temperature derangements
- Hyperglycemia

- Diaphragmatic pressure which can cause respiratory compromise
- Pleural effusions
- Visceral herniation or perforation

**Contraindications to PD:**

- Recent abdominal surgery
- Abdominal adhesions
- Peritonitis

# Electrolyte Imbalances

## Sodium

**Functions:**

- Regulates total body water
- Transmission of nerve impulses
- Regulation of acid-base balance
- Muscle contraction/ cellular depolarization

### Hypernatremia $Na^+ > 145$ mEq/L

**Causes:**

- Dehydration
- Excess administration of NaCl or $NaHCO_3$
- Hypertonic enteral feedings

**Symptoms:**

- Thirst, tachycardia, hypotension, restless, irritable, lethargy, muscle weakness, flushed skin, oliguria (with dehydration)
- May also see increased hematocrit (hemo-concentrated)
- Increased chloride
    - Often > 106 mEq/L

- Increased serum osmolality
- Increased urine specific gravity due to concentrated urine in dehydration
  - Often > 1.025
- Decreased urine $Na^+$
  - May also see ↑ in absence of dehydration

**Treatment:**

- Fluid hydration
- Free $H_2O$
- Diuretics (to remove sodium)—if appropriate for cause
  - Do **not** use if dehydrated

## Hyponatremia—$Na^+$ < 130 mEq/L

**Causes:**

- Excess $H_2O$ or $Na^+$ depletion
- Water retention
- Dehydration
- NG tube suction
- SIADH—dilutional hyponatremia
- Diarrhea
- Intestinal surgery
- DKA

**Symptoms:**

- Neuro changes, headache, confusion, coma, death
- Anxiety, weakness, abdominal cramping, seizures, hypotension, tachycardia, shock

**Treatment:**

**When treating hyponatremia, it's important to identify the patient's intravascular volume status:**

1) Water retention/Hypervolemia
   - Diuretics & sodium replacement may be administered

2) Euvolemia

- You may only give sodium replacement

3) Hypovolemia

- You may only give sodium replacement
- Slow $Na^+$ correction!!!!
  - No more than 8 - 12 mEq/day
- $Na^+$ Phosphate 1 – 2 mmol/hour over 3 – 4 hours
- Hypertonic saline
  - 2% or 3% infusion
- $Na^+$ tabs

## Potassium

- Normal $K^+$ levels: 3.5 – 5.0 mEq/L
- 98% intracellular, 2% extracellular
- $Na^+/K^+$ pump—maintains normal cell volume & electro-neutrality of the cell membrane

### Functions of K+:

- Transmission of nerve impulses
- Intracellular osmolality
- Enzymatic reactions
- Acid-base balance
- Myocardial, skeletal & smooth muscle contractility

### Potassium Regulation

- Kidneys—Primary excretory source
  - So efficient rarely have elevation in normal renal function
  - In the presence of aldosterone, $K^+$ is excreted by the renal tubules
- Intestines—excrete $K^+$

# Hypokalemia: $K^+ < 3.5$ mEq/L

## Causes:

- » Increased loss
- » GI: Vomiting, NGT suctioning
  - Aggravated by metabolic alkalosis
- » Diarrhea, fistula, ileostomy
- » Excessive urinary loss
  - Hyperaldosterone states, thiazide diuretics, amphotericin, gentamycin, cisplatin
- » Inadequate intake
- » Anorexia, ETOH
- » Magnesium depletion
- » Insulin

## Symptoms:

- » Clinical presentation—develop symptoms when $K^+ < 3.0$ mEq/L
- » Cardiovascular irritability
  - Ventricular irritability (PVCs) $K^+ < 3.2$
- » Ventricular fibrillation
- » Depressed ST segment
- » Development of a u-wave
- » Prolonged QT interval
- » Potentates digoxin activity
- » Muscle cramping
- » If the potassium is **LO**w, it causes Alka-**LO**-sis
  - 0.1 unit ↑ in pH, causes ↓ $K^+$ by 0.4 mEq/L

## Treatment:

- » Replace $K^+$
- » Oral supplements or increased dietary intake when possible
- » IV - Standard dose 10 - 20 mEq over 1 - 2 hours
  - Central line administration preferred
  - Dilute if giving through a peripheral IV
- » Eliminate or treat conditions that promote $K^+$ shifts (i.e. alkalosis)
- » Ensure adequate renal function

## Hyperkalemia - $K^+ > 5.5$ mEq

### Causes:

- » Renal failure (~75% of all cases)
    - Inability of renal tubules to excrete $K^+$
- » Acidosis
- » Decreased cardiac output
- » Elderly taking $K^+$ sparing diuretics
- » Severe trauma & burns (muscle damage)
- » Infection
- » Addison's disease
- » Increased consumption of table salt or antacids

### Symptoms:

- » Nausea & vomiting
- » Diarrhea
- » Tingling skin
- » Numbness in hands & feet
- » Flaccid paralysis
- » Apathy, confusion

### Cardiac symptoms:

- » Tall tented symmetrical T waves ($K^+ > 6.5$)
- » Widened QRS, prolonged PR, widened P wave ($K^+ > 8.0$)
- » Decreased automaticity ($K^+$ 10 - 11.0)
- » P waves may disappear
- » QRS merges with T to form sine wave
- » Asystole or ventricular fibrillation
- » Decreased strength of cardiac contraction

### Treatment:

- » Emergency (move potassium):
  - Regular Insulin IV push
    - Dextrose if normal or low glucose to prevent hypoglycemia
  - Nebulized albuterol
    - Onset ~15 min., duration about 15 – 90 min.
  - $NaHCO_3$—not as efficient as insulin
  - Calcium chloride
    - Cardiac protectant; no effect on $K^+$ levels
- » Remove potassium:
  - Dialysis
  - Loop diuretics
  - Sodium polystyrene sulfonate (Kayexalate)
    - Dose 15 grams 1 - 4 doses/ day
    - 24 hours to correct
    - Shouldn't be used for emergent treatment

## Magnesium

- » Normal level 1.5 – 2.5 mEq/L

### Functions:

- » Neuromuscular transmission
- » Cardiac contraction
- » Activation of enzymes for cellular metabolism
- » Active transport at the cellular level
- » Transmission of hereditary info.

## Hypomagnesemia - $Mg^{++} < 1.4$ mEq/L

### Causes:

- » Increased excretion
  - NG suctioning, diarrhea, fistulas
  - Diuretics: blocks $Na^+$ reabsorption
  - Osmotic diuresis
  - Antibiotics & anti-neoplastics
- » Hypercalcemia, hypokalemia
- » Decreased intake
- » Chronic alcoholism

- Malabsorption
- Acute pancreatitis

## Symptoms:

- CV: Tachycardia, depressed ST segment
- Torsades de Pointes! Caused by prolonged QT!
  - Polymorphic ventricular tachycardia
- PACs & PVCs
- Hypotension
- Increased risk for digoxin toxicity
- Coronary artery spasm
- Neuromuscular
  - Twitching, paresthesia, cramps, muscle tremors
  - + Chvostek & Trousseau's signs
    - Twitching of face or hand
- CNS: mentation changes, seizures
- Assess for hypokalemia

## Treatment:

- Assess renal function
  - Reduce $Mg^{++}$ replacement if renal dysfunction
- ↑ $Mg^{++}$ intake
- Dietary: diet or PO supplementation
  - Add to IV or TPN
- $MgSO_4$ 1 - 2 grams IV over 60 minutes, <u>emergency</u> give over 1 - 2 minutes
  - Give slowly if it's not an emergency
  - Monitor BP & airway when administering magnesium!
  - Can get hypotensive & flushed with $Mg^{++}$
- Monitor neurological status
- Monitor $K^{+}$ & $Ca^{++}$
- Follow serial magnesium levels

## Hypermagnesemia - $Mg^{++}$ > 2.5 mEq/L

### Causes:

» Decreased excretion from renal failure is the most common

» Can also see in acidosis, DKA

### Symptoms:

» 3 - 5 mEq/L Peripheral dilation, facial flushing, hypotension

» 4 - 7 mEq/L Drowsiness, lethargy

» When $Mg^{++}$ is elevated, patients get the "Mag Drag"! (Lethargy, drowsy)

### Treatment:

» ↑ excretion of $Mg^{++}$ by using fluids & diuretics

## Hypocalcemia—$Ca^{++}$ < 8.5

» Follow ionized (active) $Ca^{++}$

- Normal: 1.1 – 1.35 mmol/L

### Causes:

» Diarrhea

» Diuretics

» Malabsorption

» Chronic renal failure

» Alkalosis; $Ca^{++}$ bound to albumin & is inactive

» Phosphate & calcium have an inverse relationship to each other!

- ↑ $PO_4$ leads to ↓ $Ca^{++}$

**Symptoms:**

- CV: Prolonged QTc, ↓BP, ↓CO, ventricular ectopy, ventricular fibrillation
- Neuromuscular: Tingling, spasms, tetany, seizures
  - Twitching, paresthesia, cramps, muscle tremors
  - + Chvostek & Trousseau's signs
- Respiratory: Bronchospasm; labored shallow breathing
- Gastrointestinal: smooth muscle hyperactivity
- Bleeding; $Ca^{++}$ needed to clot
- Safety: confusion & seizures
- Muscle cramps can precede tetany

**Treatment:**

- Administer calcium

## Hypophosphatemia—$PO_4$ < 2.5 mg/dL

- Necessary for cellular energy
- Tissue catabolism: ↑ use in tissue repair

**Causes:**

- Decreased intake
- ETOH
- Small bowel disease
- Increased elimination
- Vomiting & diarrhea
- Use of phosphate binding antacids
- Increased urinary losses: osmotic diuresis, thiazide diuretics
- Increased utilization
- Intracellular shifts
- Alkalosis (respiratory)
- Refeeding syndrome
  - See when patient has been NPO & nutrition is restarted

### Symptoms: (secondary to decreases in ATP & 2,3 DPG)

» Acute:

- Confusion, seizures, coma
- Chest pain due to poor oxygenation of the myocardium
- Numbness & tingling of the fingers, circumoral region
- Incoordination
- Speech difficulty
- Weakness of respiratory muscles

» Chronic:

- Memory loss, lethargy
- Bone pain
- Hypomagnesemia

### Treatment:

» Identification & elimination of the cause

» ↑ dietary intake of phosphate

» Oral or IV phosphate supplements

- $K^+$ phosphate
- $Na^+$ phosphate

## Hyperphosphatemia—$PO_4$ > 4.5 mg/dL

### Causes:

» Increased intake from phosphate containing antacids

» Decreased excretion - renal failure

» Transcellular shifts

» Respiratory acidosis, intracellular release

» Cell lysis of RBC, skeletal muscle or tumor cells

## Symptoms:

- Rebound hypocalcemia
- Phosphate binds with free calcium & ionized serum calcium falls
- Ectopic disposition of Ca-$PO_4$
- Anorexia, nausea, vomiting
- Muscle weakness, hyperreflexia, tetany
- Tachycardia
- $\uparrow PO_4 = \downarrow Ca^{++}$

## Treatment:

- Identification & elimination of cause
- Use of aluminum, magnesium or calcium gels or antacids: binds phosphorus in the gut
- Diet low in phosphorus
- Avoid meats, fish, poultry, milk, whole grains, seeds, nuts, eggs, dried beans
- Dialysis therapy
- Acetazolamide stimulated urinary $PO_4$ excretion

| Electrolyte Imbalances & Effect on Acid/Base | |
|---|---|
| **Acidosis** | **Alkalosis** |
| Hyperkalemia | Hypokalemia |
| Hypermagnesemia | Hypomagnesemia |
| Hyperchloremia | Hypochloremia |
| Hypercalcemia | Hypocalcemia |
| Hyperphosphatemia | Hypophosphatemia |

A quick little rhyme to remember how electrolyte derangements affect acid/base:

If your electrolytes are **LO**w you'll see alka**LO**sis

If you drop **acid**, you'll get **high**!

You can do it!

# Synergy Review

## AACN Test Plan for the Professional Caring & Ethical Practice portion of the PCCN® Exam

- Advocacy/Moral Agency
- Caring Practices
- Response to Diversity
- Facilitation of Learning
- Collaboration
- Systems Thinking
- Clinical Inquiry

Note: For this section I listed "big picture" ideas to keep in mind. I recommend doing practice questions to apply many of these concepts.

# Advocacy & Moral Agency

- Working on another's behalf & representing concerns of patients, families & nursing staff (reference: AACN Synergy Model definition)
- Respecting patient's rights, beliefs & values

### Basic rights:

- Informed decision making
- Education on disease process, treatments, plan of care
- Respect & honor patient's wishes & choices
- For healthcare providers to advocate & speak up on behalf of our patients
- Privacy of information

## Multidisciplinary plan of care

- Involves the care team (providers, nursing, respiratory, PT, OT, nutrition, social work) to set comprehensive expectations of the trajectory of care for the patient

### Includes:

- Medications
- Tests
- Treatments
- Discharge needs

### Benefits of a multidisciplinary approach:

- Reduced length of stay
- Better outcomes
- Better continuity of care
- Reduced costs
- Improved communication with the patient, family & teams

## Advance Directives

» Used as a way for patients to identify their wishes at the end of life
  - They should be honored regardless of opposing family opinions

» Should identify a decision-maker if patient is incapacitated & unable to make decisions

» Consider Palliative Care consult if appropriate

» Spiritual care to meet religious needs of patient & family

» Facilitate any rituals the patient/family are requesting at end of life

» Ensure comfort
  - Outline plan with family/loved ones

**Other thoughts:**

» When communicating, always be honest

» Do not contract with family to be secretive about the patient's diagnosis

» Do not withhold information from the patient

» Always maintain confidentiality

» Use open communication
  - Ask "What is your understanding of the situation, disease state or treatment plan"?

» Keep the patient safe

» Resolve ethical & clinical concerns in a non-confrontational manner

» Consult the Ethics Committee if unable to come to resolution

## Core Patient Characteristics and Nurse Competencies as Defined in the Synergy Model

| **Advocacy and Moral Agency** | **Working on another's behalf and representing the concerns of the patient/family and nursing staff; serving as a moral agent in identifying and helping to resolve ethical and clinical concerns within and outside the clinical setting** |
|---|---|
| Level 1 | Works on behalf of patient; self-assesses personal values; aware of ethical conflicts/issues that may surface in clinical setting; makes ethical/moral decisions based on rules; represents patient when patient cannot represent self; aware of patients' rights |
| Level 3 | Works on behalf of patient and family; considers patient values and incorporates in care, even when differing from personal values; supports colleagues in ethical and clinical issues; moral decision-making can deviate from rules; demonstrates give and take with patient's family, allowing them to speak/represent themselves when possible; aware of patient and family rights |
| Level 5 | Works on behalf of patient, family and community; advocates from patient/family perspective, whether similar to or different from personal values; advocates ethical conflict and issues from patient/family perspective; suspends rules—patient and family drive moral decision-making; empowers the patient and family to speak for/represent themselves; achieves mutuality within patient/professional relationships |

Data from: American Association of Critical-Care Nurses. The AACN Synergy Model for Patient Care. Aliso Viejo, CA: AACN. https://www.aacn.org/~/media/aacn-website/nursing-excellence/standards/aacnsynergymodelforpatientcare.pdf?la=en Accessed January 26, 2020

# Caring Practices

- » Minimize safety risks to the patient
  - Communicate & speak up immediately if there is a risk or safety issue!
- » Ensure the environment is safe & comfortable for the patient
- » Ensure patient understands the plan of care
- » Identify what the patient and/or family sees as a priority in their plan of care
- » Identify a spokesperson to contact with updates
- » Ensure families are updated on the patient's status
- » Goal is always to develop trust with family
- » Assess the families coping needs & support them
- » Families are at risk for PTSD as well as patients
- » Make sure the patient & family understands expectations around visiting policies
  - How many people can visit at one time?
  - Age restrictions?
  - Is there flexibility?
- » The ideal situation/policy is open visitation tailored to the patient's wants & needs
- » Consider providing written information regarding visiting policies
  - Include unit routines
  - Shift change expectations/rules
- » Family presence during resuscitation & high risk procedures is widely accepted across the country
- » If family is present during CPR, ensure someone can stay with them for support (i.e. spiritual care, a nurse)
- » Keep the environment quiet
  - Control lights & noise as much as possible
  - Promote sleep hygiene
  - Provide eye masks & ear plugs
  - Adjust nuisance alarms from monitors
- » Consider alternative therapies as appropriate
  - Pet therapy, music therapy, aromatherapy, massage, acupuncture

## Core Patient Characteristics & Nurse Competencies as Defined in the Synergy Model

| Caring Practices | Nursing activities that create a compassionate, supportive and therapeutic environment for patients and staff, with the aim of promoting comfort and healing and preventing unnecessary suffering. Includes, but is not limited to, vigilance, engagement and responsiveness of caregivers, including family and healthcare personnel |
|---|---|
| Level 1 | Focuses on the usual and customary needs of the patient; no anticipation of future needs; bases care on standards and protocols; maintains a safe physical environment; acknowledges death as a potential outcome |
| Level 3 | Responds to subtle patient and family changes; engages with the patient as a unique patient in a compassionate manner; recognizes and tailors caring practices to the individuality of patient and family; domesticates the patient's and family's environment; recognizes that death may be an acceptable outcome |
| Level 5 | Has astute awareness and anticipates patient and family changes and needs; fully engaged with and sensing how to stand alongside the patient, family and community; caring practices follow the patient and family lead; anticipates hazards and avoids them, and promotes safety throughout patient's and family's transitions along the healthcare continuum; orchestrates the process that ensures patient's/family's comfort and concerns surrounding issues of death and dying are met |

Data from: American Association of Critical-Care Nurses. The AACN Synergy Model for Patient Care. Aliso Viejo, CA: AACN. https://www.aacn.org/~/media/aacn-website/nursing-excellence/standards/aacnsynergy-modelforpatientcare.pdf?la=en Accessed January 26, 2020

# Response to Diversity

- Make every effort to meet the ethical, religious & cultural needs of your patient
- Cultural sensitivity—be aware of differences that may impact clinical care
- Incorporate the patient's values into care as much as possible
- Avoid stereotypes of cultures & race
- Modify care to meet the patient's needs
- Pain may be expressed differently based on culture
- Maintain patient privacy
- Consider dietary needs based on cultural differences (i.e. vegetarian, no beef or pork)

**Core Patient Characteristics & Nurse Competencies as Defined in the Synergy Model**

| Response to Diversity | The sensitivity to recognize, appreciate and incorporate differences into the provision of care; differences may include, but are not limited to, cultural differences, spiritual beliefs, gender, race, ethnicity, lifestyle, socioeconomic status, age and values |
|---|---|
| Level 1 | Assesses cultural diversity; provides care based on own belief system; learns the culture of the healthcare environment |
| Level 3 | Inquires about cultural differences and considers their impact on care; accommodates personal and professional differences in the plan of care; helps patient/family understand the culture of the healthcare system |
| Level 5 | Responds to, anticipates and integrates cultural differences into patient/family care; appreciates and incorporates differences, including alternative therapies, into care; tailors healthcare culture, to the extent possible, to meet the diverse needs and strengths of the patient/family |

Data from: American Association of Critical-Care Nurses. The AACN Synergy Model for Patient Care. Aliso Viejo, CA: AACN. https://www.aacn.org/~/media/aacn-website/nursing-excellence/standards/aacnsynergy-modelforpatientcare.pdf?la=en Accessed January 26, 2020

# Facilitation of Learning

## Staff Educational Needs

- » If you have not been trained to care for certain patients or devices/treatments they are receiving, you should not accept that assignment or agree to cover for breaks
- » Notify the charge nurse immediately to be assigned to a different patient
- » You must meet the competencies to care for patients with specialized needs (i.e. dialysis)

## Patient & Family Educational Needs

- » Teach back method—have them show you how to do a skill vs. telling them how to do it
- » Provide ongoing education if needed
- » Provide episodic education based on learning needs
- » Do not wait until discharge to provide all teaching at once
- » Repeat & reinforce the information & assesses for knowledge deficits
- » Specialty consults for specific educational needs (i.e. heart failure, diabetic education)
- » Identify barriers to learning (i.e. cognitive, language) & re-strategize educational plans
- » If there is a language barrier, consult a medical interpreter
    - Families or friends should not be used to interpret medical information
- » Avoid medical jargon & terminology as much as possible

**Core Patient Characteristics and Nurse Competencies as Defined in the Synergy Model**

| Facilitation of Learning | The ability to facilitate learning for patients/families, nursing staff, other members of the healthcare team and community; includes both formal and informal facilitation of learning |
|---|---|
| Level 1 | Follows planned educational programs; sees patient/family education as a separate task from delivery of care; provides data without seeking to assess patient's readiness or understanding; has limited knowledge of the totality of the educational needs; focuses on a nurse's perspective; sees the patient as a passive recipient |
| Level 3 | Adapts planned educational programs; begins to recognize and integrate different ways of teaching into delivery of care; incorporates patient's understanding into practice; sees the overlapping of educational plans from different healthcare providers' perspectives; begins to see the patient as having input into goals; begins to see individualism |
| Level 5 | Creatively modifies or develops patient/family education programs; integrates patient/family education throughout delivery of care; evaluates patient's understanding by observing behavior changes related to learning; is able to collaborate and incorporate all healthcare providers' and educational plans into the patient/family educational program; sets patient-driven goals for education; sees patient/family as having choices and consequences that are negotiated in relation to education |

Data from: American Association of Critical-Care Nurses. The AACN Synergy Model for Patient Care. Aliso Viejo, CA: AACN. https://www.aacn.org/~/media/aacn-website/nursing-excellence/standards/aacnsynergymodelforpatientcare.pdf?la=en Accessed January 26, 2020

# Collaboration

- Make referrals as needed for other multidisciplinary services
  - Example: If you patient is high risk for skin breakdown, consult with Physical Therapy & Nutrition
- Include family as much as appropriate in planning & patient care
- Include patients & families in multidisciplinary rounds as much as possible
- Prepare patients & families for transitions in care as early as possible
  - Transfer to another unit or facility
- If the patient is transferring to another unit or facility, encourage the family to tour the new location prior to transfer
  - This may reduce fear & anxiety
  - Consider having the unit charge nurse or manager meet the patient & family prior to discharge
- If discharging, assess resources available for patient
  - Consult social work or appropriate groups for gaps in resources

## Core Patient Characteristics and Nurse Competencies as Defined in the Synergy Model

| **Collaboration** | **Working with others (e.g., patients, families, healthcare providers) in a way that promotes/encourages each person's contributions toward achieving optimal/realistic patient/family goals; involves intra- and inter-disciplinary work with colleagues and community** |
|---|---|
| Level 1 | Willing to be taught, coached and/or mentored; participates in team meetings and discussions regarding patient care and/or practice issues; open to various team members' contributions |
| Level 3 | Seeks opportunities to be taught, coached and/or mentored; elicits others' advice and perspectives; initiates and participates in team meetings and discussions regarding patient care and/or practice issues; recognizes and suggests various team members' participation |
| Level 5 | Seeks opportunities to teach, coach and mentor and to be taught, coached and mentored; facilitates active involvement and complementary contributions of others in team meetings and discussions regarding patient care and/or practice issues; involves/recruits diverse resources when appropriate to optimize patient outcomes |

Data from: American Association of Critical-Care Nurses. The AACN Synergy Model for Patient Care. Aliso Viejo, CA: AACN. https://www.aacn.org/~/media/aacn-website/nursing-excellence/standards/aacnsynergy-modelforpatientcare.pdf?la=en Accessed January 26, 2020

# Systems Thinking

## Patient Safety

- If a mistake is made, do not try to cover it up
- Talk to the patient & family about what happened
- Apologize for the mistake
- Explain the plan for follow up
- If a mistake is made, always assess for system issues
- Consider participating in a hospital committee to better understand system issues
- Maintain a non-punitive environment to support healthcare providers

## General rules:

- Avoid unapproved abbreviations
- Always use 2 person identifiers
    - Name, Medical Record Number, DOB

**Core Patient Characteristics and Nurse Competencies as Defined in the Synergy Model**

| **Systems Thinking** | **Body of knowledge and tools that allow the nurse to manage whatever environmental and system resources exist for the patient/family and staff, within or across healthcare and non-healthcare systems** |
|---|---|
| Level 1 | Uses a limited array of strategies; limited outlook—sees the pieces or components; does not recognize negotiation as an alternative; sees patient and family within the isolated environment of the unit; sees self as key resource |
| Level 3 | Develops strategies based on needs and strengths of patient/family; able to make connections within components; sees opportunity to negotiate, but may not have strategies; developing a view of the patient/family transition process; recognizes how to obtain resources beyond self |
| Level 5 | Develops, integrates and applies a variety of strategies that are driven by the needs and strengths of the patient/family; global or holistic outlook—sees the whole rather than the pieces; knows when and how to negotiate and navigate through the system on behalf of patients and families; anticipates needs of patients and families as they move through the healthcare system; utilizes untapped and alternative resources as necessary |

Data from: American Association of Critical-Care Nurses. The AACN Synergy Model for Patient Care. Aliso Viejo, CA: AACN. https://www.aacn.org/~/media/aacn-website/nursing-excellence/standards/aacnsynergy-modelforpatientcare.pdf?la=en Accessed January 26, 2020

# Clinical Inquiry

## Evidence-Based Practice (EBP)

- Understanding of what the best, most reliable evidence is to provide a standard of care for patients
- Don't practice on the idea of "That's the way we've always done it"
- If there is a need for a change in practice:
  - Collaborate with multidisciplinary team
  - Conduct a literature review
  - Randomized-controlled trials would be highest level of evidence
  - Systematic reviews & meta-analysis are very helpful
  - Consider national practice guidelines from professional organizations (i.e. American Heart Association, Surviving Sepsis Campaign)
- Establish a unit-based council
- Create an environment of inquiry

### Core Patient Characteristics and Nurse Competencies as Defined in the Synergy Model

| **Clinical Judgment** | **Clinical reasoning, which includes clinical decision-making, critical thinking and a global grasp of the situation, coupled with nursing skills acquired through a process of integrating formal and informal experiential knowledge and evidence-based guidelines** |
|---|---|
| Level 1 | Collects basic-level data; follows algorithms, decision trees and protocols with all populations and is uncomfortable deviating from them; matches formal knowledge with clinical events to make decisions; questions the limits of one's ability to make clinical decisions and delegates the decision-making to other clinicians; includes extraneous detail |
| Level 3 | Collects and interprets complex patient data; makes clinical judgments based on an immediate grasp of the whole picture for common or routine patient populations; recognizes patterns and trends that may predict the direction of illness; recognizes limits and seeks appropriate help; focuses on key elements of case, while sorting out extraneous details |

| | |
|---|---|
| Level 5 | Synthesizes and interprets multiple, sometimes conflicting, sources of data; makes judgment based on an immediate grasp of the whole picture, unless working with new patient populations; uses past experiences to anticipate problems; helps patient and family see the "big picture"; recognizes the limits of clinical judgment and seeks multidisciplinary collaboration and consultation with comfort; recognizes and responds to the dynamic situation |

Data from: American Association of Critical-Care Nurses. The AACN Synergy Model for Patient Care. Aliso Viejo, CA: AACN. https://www.aacn.org/~/media/aacn-website/nursing-excellence/standards/aacnsynergy-modelforpatientcare.pdf?la=en Accessed January 26, 2020

## Core Patient Characteristics and Nurse Competencies as Defined in the Synergy Model

| **Clinical Inquiry** | **The ongoing process of questioning and evaluating practice and providing informed practice; creating practice changes through research utilization and experiential learning** |
|---|---|
| Level 1 | Follows standards and guidelines; implements clinical changes and research-based practices developed by others; recognizes the need for further learning to improve patient care; recognizes obvious changing patient situation (e.g., deterioration, crisis); needs and seeks help to identify patient problem |
| Level 3 | Questions appropriateness of policies and guidelines; questions current practice; seeks advice, resources or information to improve patient care; begins to compare and contrast possible alternatives |
| Level 5 | Improves, deviates from or individualizes standards and guidelines for particular patient situations or populations; questions and/or evaluates current practice based on patients' responses, review of the literature, research and education/learning; acquires knowledge and skills needed to address questions arising in practice and improve patient care; (The domains of clinical judgment and clinical inquiry converge at the expert level; they cannot be separated) |

Data from: American Association of Critical-Care Nurses. The AACN Synergy Model for Patient Care. Aliso Viejo, CA: AACN. https://www.aacn.org/~/media/aacn-website/nursing-excellence/standards/aacnsynergy-modelforpatientcare.pdf?la=en Accessed January 26, 2020

## Legal/Ethical Principles

### Beneficence:

- The action that is done for the benefit of others
- Beneficent actions can be taken to help prevent or remove harms or to simply improve the situation of others

### Nonmaleficence:

- "Do no harm"
- Refrain from providing ineffective treatments or acting with malice toward patients
  - Offers little useful guidance to physicians since many beneficial therapies also have serious risks
- Pertinent ethical issue is whether the benefits outweigh the burdens

### Veracity:

- Principle of truth telling, & it is grounded in respect for persons & the concept of autonomy

### Justice:

- The fair distribution of benefits & burdens

**Paternalism:**

» What is best for patients may affect the decisions they make about their patient's diagnosis, prognosis or therapy

» The nurse may choose to withhold information from the patient & family members

» The interference with a person's liberty of action justified by reason referring exclusively to the welfare of the person being coerced

**Fidelity:**

» Dedication, loyalty, truthfulness, advocacy & fairness to patients

**Confidentiality:**

» The obligation of professionals who have access to patient records or communication to hold that information in confidence

**Utilitarianism:**

» To promote the greatest good that is possible in situations

You can do it!

## Core Patient Characteristics and Nurse Competencies as Defined in the Synergy Model

| Patient Characteristics | Description |
|---|---|
| **Resiliency** | **The capacity to return to a restorative level of functioning using compensatory/coping mechanisms; the ability to bounce back quickly after an insult** |
| Level 1—Minimally resilient | Unable to mount a response; failure of compensatory/coping mechanisms; minimal reserves; brittle |
| Level 3—Moderately resilient | Able to mount a moderate response; able to initiate some degree of compensation; moderate reserves |
| Level 5—Highly resilient | Able to mount and maintain a response; intact compensatory/coping mechanisms; strong reserves; endurance |
| **Vulnerability** | **Susceptibility to actual or potential stressors that may adversely affect patient outcomes** |
| Level 1—Highly vulnerable | Susceptible; unprotected, fragile |
| Level 3—Moderately vulnerable | Somewhat susceptible; somewhat protected |
| Level 5—Minimally vulnerable | Safe; out of the woods; protected, not fragile |
| **Stability** | **The ability to maintain a steady-state equilibrium** |
| Level 1—Minimally stable | Labile; unstable; unresponsive to therapies; high risk of death |
| Level 3—Moderately stable | Able to maintain steady state for limited period of time; some responsiveness to therapies |
| Level 5—Highly stable | Constant; responsive to therapies; low risk of death |
| **Complexity** | **The intricate entanglement of two or more systems (e.g., body, family, therapies)** |
| Level 1—Highly complex | Intricate; complex patient/family dynamics; ambiguous/vague; atypical presentation |
| Level 3—Moderately complex | Moderately involved patient/family dynamics |
| Level 5—Minimally complex | Straightforward; routine patient/family dynamics; simple/clear cut; typical presentation |

| **Resource availability** | **Extent of resources (e.g., technical, fiscal, personal, psychological and social) the patient/family/ community bring to the situation** |
|---|---|
| Level 1—Few resources | Necessary knowledge and skills not available; necessary financial support not available; minimal personal/psychological supportive resources; few social systems resources |
| Level 3—Moderate resources | Limited knowledge and skills available; limited financial support available; limited personal/psychological supportive resources; limited social systems resources |
| Level 5—Many resources | Extensive knowledge and skills available and accessible; financial resources readily available; strong personal/ psychological supportive resources; strong social systems resources |
| **Participation in care** | **Extent to which patient/family engages in aspects of care** |
| Level 1—No participation | Patient and family unable or unwilling to participate in care |
| Level 3—Moderate level of participation | Patient and family need assistance in care |
| Level 5—Full participation | Patient and family fully able to participate in care |
| **Participation in decision-making** | **Extent to which patient/family engages in decision-making** |
| Level 1—No participation | Patient and family have no capacity for decision-making; requires surrogacy |
| Level 3—Moderate level of participation | Patient and family have limited capacity; seeks input/ advice from others in decision-making |
| Level 5—Full participation | Patient and family have capacity, and makes decision for self |
| **Predictability** | **A characteristic that allows one to expect a certain course of events or course of illness** |
| Level 1—Not predictable | Uncertain; uncommon patient population/illness; unusual or unexpected course; does not follow critical pathway, or no critical pathway developed |
| Level 3—Moderately predictable | Wavering; occasionally noted patient population/illness |
| Level 5—Highly predictable | Certain; common patient population/illness; usual and expected course; follows critical pathway |

Source: AACN

# About the author...

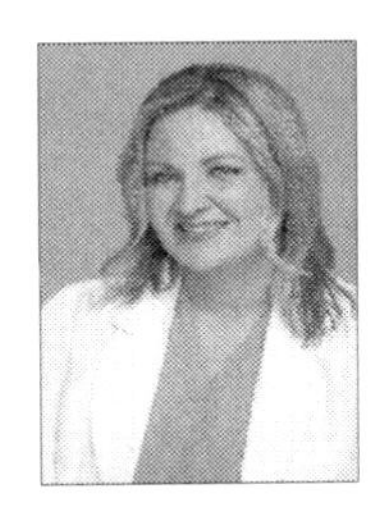

Nicole Kupchik has practiced as a Critical Care nurse for over twenty-five years. She obtained a Nursing Degree from Purdue University in 1993 and a Master of Nursing from the University of Washington in 2008.

Nicole's nursing career began in the Chicago area. From 1995 to 1998, she journeyed across the United States as a traveling nurse, after which she landed in Seattle. Her first job in Seattle was in the Cardiothoracic Intensive Care Unit (5 SE) at the University of Washington. In 2001, she began working at Harborview Medical Center—a change that spurred an interest in resuscitation.

Shortly thereafter, Nicole was part of a multidisciplinary team that was one of the first in the United States to implement therapeutic hypothermia after cardiac arrest. As part of this effort, Nicole was responsible for protocol development and has published numerous papers on this topic.

In 2008, Nicole was part of a team that implemented a formalized Sepsis program at Harborview Medical Center. The program resulted in a reduction in mortality, hospital length of stay and a significant cost avoidance. She collaborated with IT specialists to develop innovative methods to electronically screen hospitalized patients in acute care units for sepsis. For this work, the program was awarded two Patient Safety & Clinical Leadership awards.

In 2002, Nicole obtained certification as a CCRN®. She admittedly attended three certification review courses before finally taking the exam! Once she passed the exam she questioned why she hesitated and lacked confidence to sit the exam. Shortly thereafter, Nicole began teaching segments of CCRN® & PCCN® certification review courses at her hospital. In 2006, she started co-teaching courses nationally.

In 2013, Nicole founded Nicole Kupchik Consulting & Education. She frequently teaches review courses nationally. Currently, she holds certification as a CCNS®, CCRN®, PCCN®, CMC® & CSC®.

Her courses are well attended and often sell out! Her wit and sense of humor make the course interesting & entertaining. Nicole has a gift of being able to break information down in a way that is really easy to understand. She hopes to instill confidence in attendees that they can do it!

## OTHER BOOKS BY NICOLE KUPCHIK

*Ace the CCRN®: You Can Do It! Practice Review Questions*

*Ace the CCRN®: You can do it! Study Guide*

*Ace the PCCN®: You Can Do It! Practice Review Questions*

*Ace the CMC®: You Can Do It! Study Guide with Practice Review Questions*

*Ace the CSC®: You Can Do It! Study Guide with Practice Review Questions*

Nicole also has online courses available for
the CCRN®, PCCN® & CMC® exams!

## FOLLOW NICOLE ON SOCIAL MEDIA:

Nicole Kupchik Consulting & Education

@nicolekupchik

YouTube Nicole Kupchik

**Podcast:** Resus10 on Apple & Stitcher

You can do it!

Made in the USA
Columbia, SC
19 October 2024